Homicide and Severe Mental Disorder

T0384826

Homicide and Severe Mental Disorder: Understanding and Prevention provides a complete picture of how severe mental disorder can be assessed in cases of homicide, and how improved understanding can impact risk reduction and prevention. Michael Farrell brings together a wide range of material including theory, research, demographic data, case examples, enquiry reports, and practical strategies, providing clear examples throughout.

Farrell draws on examples of homicide representing a great challenge to both comprehension and prevention – cases that have sometimes provoked media criticism of public policy and services and have aroused public anxiety. In seeking fuller understanding, the book takes an overview of severe mental disorder, homicide, and prevention, before introducing the approach of Situational Crime Prevention and related theory and discussing demographic features of perpetrators and victims. Turning to prevention, the text examines examples of research into homicides perpetrated by individuals with severe mental disorder. Insights from Situational Crime Prevention are applied to selected cases, and a wider view is then taken looking at the criminological features of means, motive, opportunity, and location. Organisational constraints and limitations of communication in services are considered, and cases illuminating the issues and challenges throughout the book are summarised in a structured end of volume glossary. As evidence and insights accumulate and cohere, they more clearly indicate preventive strategies.

Homicide and Severe Mental Disorder will be of great interest to students, researchers, and teachers in psychiatry, psychology, and criminology, health and mental health professionals, criminal justice personnel, and those working with individuals with severe mental disorder.

Michael Farrell has written extensively for medical, legal, and police publications. He is the author of *Psychosis Under Discussion* (Routledge) and his textbooks on provision for individuals with mental disorders are translated into Asian, Middle Eastern, and European languages.

This volume provides a masterful combination of theory, research, practice, and policy to focus on how homicides resulting from serious mental disorder may be prevented. A must read for all students of mental disorder and its relationship to violence.

Prof Graeme Newman, University at Albany – State
University of New York, USA

Discussing a profoundly serious topic which has many misconceptions surrounding it, this book is excellent reading for anybody who deals with criminal justice and mental health. I recommend it strongly.

Dr Walid Sarhan MD, FRCPsych, IDFAPA,
Chief Editor *Arab Journal of Psychiatry*

This book is aimed at a broad readership who will be interested in this topic, including students, researchers, and teachers in criminology, psychology, and psychiatry, criminal justice personnel, and mental health professionals. Furthermore, homicide and serious mental disorder are universal to all cultures and societies and therefore this book will attract a wide international readership.

Prof Jenny Shaw, National Confidential Inquiry into
Suicide and Safety in Mental Health, The
University of Manchester, UK

Homicide and Severe Mental Disorder

Understanding and Prevention

Michael Farrell

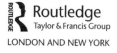
Routledge
Taylor & Francis Group

LONDON AND NEW YORK

First published 2021
by Routledge
2 Park Square, Milton Park, Abingdon, Oxon OX14 4RN

and by Routledge
605 Third Avenue, New York, NY 10158

Routledge is an imprint of the Taylor & Francis Group, an informa business

British Library Cataloguing-in-Publication Data
A catalogue record for this book is available from the British Library

Library of Congress Cataloging-in-Publication Data
A catalog record has been requested for this book

ISBN: 978-1-032-00099-2 (hbk)
ISBN: 978-1-032-00097-8 (pbk)
ISBN: 978-1-003-17272-7 (ebk)

DOI: 10.4324/9781003172727

Typeset in Times New Roman
by Taylor & Francis Books

Contents

Tables

Preface

Mental disorder and homicide are complex and worldwide issues. In writing *Homicide and Severe Mental Disorder: Understanding and Prevention* I have integrated ideas and information from many sources to extend understanding and identify approaches to prevention. Doing this has involved drawing on sources of research, case studies, investigative reports, and other material from Europe, the United States of America, Australia, New Zealand, Singapore, and elsewhere. Reflecting this international breadth, it has been an asset to have the support of colleagues (mentioned in the acknowledgements) from the United States of America, the United Kingdom, Australia, and Jordan who have commented on chapters of the book.

In this context, I hope that this volume is useful to those working in professional areas where the issues covered are important, and that it also engages others wishing to gain a clearer picture of the challenges involved. I would be happy to receive comments and suggestions that might inform any future editions at the following e-mail address:

drmjfarrell@bulldog1870.plus.com

Michael Farrell
Herefordshire, UK

Acknowledgements

I am grateful to friends and colleagues for commenting on various chapters.
Dr Clare Allely, Reader in Forensic Psychology, University of Salford, UK.
Dr Alison Baird, National Confidential Inquiry into Suicide and Safety in
Mental Health, University of Manchester, UK. The Reverend Susan Bull, Chair
of the mental health charity *Love Me Love My Mind*. Dr Andrew Butterfill MD,
St Christopher's Winter Shelter, Hereford, UK. Prof. Helen Herrman, Professor
of Psychiatry and Director of Research, Orygen University of Melbourne, Australia. Dr Richard Hough, Criminology and Criminal Justice Administration
and Law, University of West Florida, US. Dr Saied Ibrahim, National Confidential Inquiry into Suicide and Safety in Mental Health, University of Manchester, UK. Professor Graeme Newman, Distinguished Professor Emeritus at
the School of Criminal Justice, University at Albany, State University of New
York. Dr Walid Sarhan, Consultant Psychiatrist and Chief Editor *Arab Journal
of Psychiatry*, Amman, Jordan. Professor Jenny Shaw, National Confidential
Inquiry into Suicide and Safety in Mental Health, University of Manchester, UK.

Shaun Kennedy at the Royal College of Psychiatrists, London kindly helped
with initial searches at the RCP library and archives. Staff at the British Library,
London gave impeccable service.

As well, I am grateful to friends who are not specialists in the areas covered in
the book whose comments helped to improve the clarity of the text so that it
might better engage an interested general reader. They are Richard Aird OBE,
John Dewhurst, Dr Michael Lafferty, John Pitt, and Gordon Springford whose
expertise variously covered engineering, education, special education, archi-
tecture, philosophy of art, and accountancy and banking.

Chapter I

Prospect

Introduction

This chapter presents examples of recent cases of homicide by individuals with
severe mental disorder (SMD) and shows how these are represented in media
coverage including popular newspapers which sometimes caricature events. It
looks at potential negative implications of public perceptions of SMD homicides
on people with mental disorders who harm no one. The chapter also considers
the importance of recognising the impact of SMD homicides on victims' families
and the local community. For the book as a whole, the aims, scope, methodol-
ogy, special features, and proposed readers are set out. Leading into the rest of
the book, an outline and structure of subsequent chapters is provided.

The impact of SMD homicides

About 7.30 am on 7 March 2013, Christine Edkins, a 16-year-old schoolgirl boarded the bus on her way to Leasowes High School, Birmingham, UK. Ascending to
the upper deck, she sat alone partway down the aisle. Another passenger, Philip
Simelane, was already seated further back. He left his seat, walked forwards as if
towards the front exit stairs then stabbed Edkins as he passed her seat. As the attack
was unexpected and random, other passengers on the upper deck did not realise
what had happened until Christina Edkins showed signs of distress by which time
Simelane had left the bus. He was arrested soon after (Reed, 2014). On at least two
occasions previously, a specialist registrar in psychiatry had insisted that Simelane
'needed in-patient treatment' but this was not made available.

In the US, Deana Laney beat to death her sons Joshua, 8, and Luke, 6, with a
rock in the yard outside her home. A member of an Assemblies of God church,
Laney had told fellow worshipers a year earlier that the world was ending, and
that God had ordered her to get her house in order. After the killing she telephoned emergency services and told them what she had done (CNN/KLTV,
2003; Falkenberg, 2003).

On 29 February 2016 outside Oktabrskoye Pole Metro Station in North
West Moscow a woman was seen holding up the severed head of a child. The

DOI: 10.4324/9781003172727-1

woman was nanny Gyulchekhra Bobokulova, the child Anastasia Meshcher-yakova, a four-year-old in her care. Years before, Bobokulova had been trea-ted in her native Ukraine for schizophrenia. After being arrested in Moscow, she told police that she was acting on Allah's orders, and that voices had prompted her to kill Anastasia (TASS, 2016).

In Maine, US, William Bruce had been diagnosed with 'paranoid schizophrenia' (schizophrenia with delusions of persecution) after a series of violent incidents. In June 2006, alone in the house with his mother Amy, he struck her with a hatchet as she sat working at her desk and deposited her body in the bathtub. He deludedly believed that she was an al Qaeda agent (Bernstein and Koppel, 2008).

When events such as these occur, they typically attract extensive news cov-erage, some of which raises questions about possible prevention.

News media coverage

News coverage of homicide and mental disorder

A *New York Times* story (Sontag, 2011) covers the killing in Boston of Ste-phanie Moulton, a 'petite, street-smart 25-year-old' by 27-year-old Deshawn James Chappell 'a schizophrenic with a violent criminal record'. Stephanie Moulton was a health worker in the group home where Deshawn Chappell was based. Prosecutors stated that Chappell, 'beat her, stabbed her repeatedly and then dumped her partially nude body in a church parking lot'.

A UK newspaper, the *Sun* (Reporter, 2013) in an article headlined, '1,200 killed by mental patients: Shock 10-year toll exposes care crisis', criticised the lack of communication between agencies as well as serious failings of community care.

A *Daily Mail On-line* article (Linning, 2015) about a 'Psycho killer' states, 'Emmanuel Kalejaiye stabbed his mother Tolu Kalejaiye more than 40 times'; 'He dressed up in women's clothing to make neighbours think she was alive'; and the case 'echoed 1960 Hitchcock film in which killer impersonated dead mother'.

The *Daily Mail* (Greenwood, Brooke and Dolan, 2016, p. 1) reporting the death of Jo Cox, a UK Member of Parliament, states that she was 'shot three times with a sawn-off shotgun and stabbed repeatedly with a foot long hunt-ing knife in frenzied attack'. The killer 'kicked, stabbed and then shot' the MP 'at almost point-blank range'. A subheading added that Jo Cox was 'brutally murdered by a loner with a history of mental illness'.

Selection of facts and descriptions

Analysis of such stories including the examples already mentioned (Farrell, 2018, pp. 125–140) shows that they are often structured to convey the seeming unfa-thomability and dramatic violence of some of these attacks. In this way, they are crafted to humanise the victim rather than the perpetrator. Perpetrators are briefly identified as being killers and psychotic. There is a 'a dangerous paranoid schizophrenic ... on trial release from a secure mental hospital', a 'cross-dressing Psycho-style killer', 'a schizophrenic with a violent criminal record', and 'a loner with a history of mental illness'. Bringing out the unpredictability of attacks showing the danger even of friends, is a report of a victim being killed by 'his schizophrenic lifelong pal'. Similarly, the normally trusted figure of a nanny is instead dangerous, sinister, and duplicitous – a 'killer nanny' or a 'hijab-wearing nanny' who 'kept her schizophrenia a secret'.

By contrast, descriptions of victims attract the reader's sympathy. Youth is foregrounded, sometimes linked to victims being of school age or even younger as with a '16 year old ... on her way to school on a bus'; a 'thirteen year old school girl', and a 'four year old girl'. Professionals who were trying to help are sympathetically identified, as with 'mental health worker Ashleigh Ewing aged 22 years'. There is also 'a prominent schizophrenia specialist' who helped patients by 'sheer force of sympathy and good will'. Conveying a death leaving innocent dependents a victim is described as a 'father of two'. While the vulnerability of age is captured with the reference to a 'mother ... aged 79 years', the defencelessness of diminutive size is indicated by a 'petite, street-smart 25-year-old'.

Details of attacks are conveyed vividly. Stabbings are linked with places that the reader might consider safe. One victim was 'stabbed to death in a park' and another 'on the doorstep of his home'. Repeated stabbing is regularly mentioned along with the expression 'frenzied' to underline the ferocity of the attack. Details of the weapon or manner of killing are provided. Accordingly, a victim was 'stabbed 17 times with a samurai sword', another 'died after being stabbed 39 times', and a mother was stabbed 'more than 40 times' in a 'frenzied attack'. A further victim was 'shot three times with a sawn-off shotgun and stabbed repeatedly with a foot-long hunting knife in a frenzied attack'. Of one victim it is stated that the attacker 'beat her, stabbed her repeatedly and then dumped her partially nude body in a church parking lot'. A mother was shot 'in the face'. The nanny who had beheaded a four-year-old girl walked the streets 'brandishing the head of the child'.

Media reports are crafted to bring disturbing events vividly to the public's attention. As such they can be over sensationalised but can also raise justified issues about prevention in seeking to hold authorities to account.

Creating prejudice towards those with mental disorders and side-lining victims' families

Where cases involving people with SMD are reported and discussed, and especially where they involve dramatic violence and/or random attacks, concern is sometimes expressed that this may provoke prejudice towards individuals with mental disorders more generally. This can lead to suggestions that accounts of the homicides do not over sensationalise events. Detailed descriptions may be seen as potentially inflammatory.

It may be pointed out that people with mental disorder are more likely to be vulnerable to violence and be the subject of attacks than they are to perpetrate violence. Researchers examining a Swedish population-based cohort found that individuals with schizophrenia were nearly twice as likely to be victims of homicide as they were to be perpetrators (Crump, Sundquist, Winkleby and Sundquist, 2013).

Also, instances of homicide and of violence generally are rare among individuals with mental disorders. Indeed, the great majority of individuals with mental disorder harm no one. A global study mentions the rarity of criminal homicide among people with psychosis, reflecting which it allocates only an indirect footnote (United Nations Office on Drugs and Crime, 2013).

An example of emphasising the rarity of SMD homicide occurs in a *Sun* newspaper story of 7 October 2013. After citing killings by people with SMD, the reporter quotes a spokesperson for MIND, a UK mental health charity, who points out that, 'Mental health is far too often spoken of in terms of aggression and violence'. He adds that 'We must remember that there are 1.2 million people in touch with mental health services – and the overwhelming majority are not hurting others'.

While such comments from mental health charities and others are protective of people with mental disorder who harm no one, they can seem to minimise the shock and grief of those directly affected by the killings. Consequently, such perspectives do not always strike a chord with the wider community. Instead of providing a context for the homicide, which is the intention, they can be seen as one sided.

Families and friends of victims killed by individuals with SMD may want to convey the trauma of the homicide by ensuring that it is described by the media and in court (as they might see it) without euphemism. In court they may feel side-lined.

A Hundred Families is a UK-based charity supporting the families of victims of a mental health homicide. Their practical guide points out, 'The court proceedings often focus on the offender and the defending lawyers will usually put forward all sorts of arguments why they should be treated leniently. The voice of the victim, and the impact their violent death has had on the family, can often be completely lost in this process.' (A Hundred Families, 2015, p. 13).

The present book aims, while examining some of the most challenging cases regarding understanding and prevention, to be neither over sensationalising nor euphemistic.

The book's main themes and objectives and its content

Homicide and Severe Mental Disorder: Understanding and Prevention has two purposes. Firstly, it lays a foundation of understanding by discussing SMD and homicide, Situational Crime Prevention, and demographic features of perpetrators and victims (such as age and gender).

Next, the book identifies preventive approaches for homicides by people with SMD. It does this through considering research assessing the risk of violence, examining recent cases including via Situational Crime Prevention, exploring criminological features such as means and location, and discussing problems with organization and communication in mental health services, the police service, and elsewhere.

Methodology and rationale

The book focuses on understanding homicide by perpetrators with SMD and developing opportunities to prevent it. In doing so, it first presents information to aid understanding by defining and discussing SMD, homicide, and prevention, and by presenting demographic data.

Next the book examines prevention from a range of perspectives. Research into homicide and SMD is reviewed with a focus on implications for prevention. Situational Crime Prevention is used to analyse a small number of cases and indicate where the theory sheds light on issues and importantly where it has limitations, and therefore what alternative responses could be. Means, motive, opportunity, and location are considered. Organisational constraints inhibiting prevention are discussed.

In illustrating preventive issues, the book refers to around 25 cases with which the reader becomes increasingly familiar. Some of these are presented as detailed case studies. In this way, the book brings together wider research into the risk of violence and homicide, detailed case studies, and broader case analysis.

The cases discussed and outlined in the book's glossary were selected according to the following criteria:

- They concern *homicides perpetrated by individuals with SMD.*
- They nearly all involve perpetrators judged *legally 'insane'* and not criminally responsible.
- They are *relatively recent* so likely more relevant to current circumstances than cases from many decades ago.
- They represent some of the *most challenging cases* to try to understand, being sometimes random, and often dramatically violent.
- They draw on *publicly available material* to which the reader can refer, and include research studies, press reports, investigative papers, and court documents often with internet links.
- They help to identify *preventive themes* for the future, indicate errors made by professional groups and authorities that *suggest lessons to be learned*, and point to *mitigating risk.*

Structure of chapters

While the book is coherent and unified in its content and tone, individual chapters are structured to be understandable as an e-book component that may have been bought separately. Each e-book chapter comprises an abstract and key words. Both e-book and print versions contain an introduction, headings, and sub-headings to guide the reader, a conclusion, suggested activities to stimulate discussion and further study, a few key texts, and a list of references with internet sources where applicable.

Proposed readers

The book uses material and examples especially from the United States and the United Kingdom but also including other countries. It is intended for:

- students, researchers, and teachers in criminology, psychology, and psychiatry.
- criminal justice personnel (police, probation services, the prison services, lawyers, and those supporting them).
- health and mental health professionals (physicians, nurses, paramedics, psychiatrists, psychiatric nurses, psychologists, social workers exercising mental health responsibilities, those working for mental health charities, and administrators).
- local authority housing officers, workers in homeless shelters, and in 'half-way houses', and others working in the community as paid employees or volunteers.

The volume concerns psychiatry and psychology, mental health, criminology, policing, probation, social work, prison services, courts, administration, and policy making.

Given the vital role of members of the local community, for example acting as volunteers, the book could be read by all of those interested in the issues discussed. To this end, advice has been sought from professionals and those directly involved, but also importantly from non-specialist members of the community. The generous support of all these people is reflected in the acknowledgements at the beginning of the book.

By good fortune, my books over the years have been read worldwide in English and in translation into Asian, Middle Eastern, and European languages. This volume is global in scope and is intended to be read internationally in countries where English is the first language, and in areas where English is widely spoken and understood, for example Scandinavia.

Outline of the remaining chapters

Part I Understanding

Chapter 2 Understanding SMD, homicide, and prevention

This chapter defines SMD and provides examples. As many such disorders involve psychotic features, the chapter describes psychosis and how it is fundamentally related to or associated with SMDs. Schizophrenia, substance/

medication-induced psychotic disorder, depressive disorder, and manic episodes are the main foci. For each of these topics is provided a definition,
diagnostic criteria, prevalence, risk factors, and a brief description of
treatment.

Next, homicide is defined, and types of homicide are discussed including
ones indicating the relationship between perpetrator and victim, like matricide. Legal understandings of insanity and tests of criminal responsibility such
as the McNaughton Rule are considered. Reference is made to instances of
homicide by perpetrators with SMD. Finally, the notion of prevention and
the reduction of homicides is discussed.

Chapter 3 Understanding Situational Crime Prevention

This chapter introduces Situational Crime Prevention (SCP), focusing on its
origins and development, features of SCP, its strategies and techniques, and
its application to homicide involving severe mental disorder. The development
of SCP is described from its origins in the study of school absconding.

Among features of SCP are its theoretical underpinnings leading to preventive suggestions, the importance of related theories, the behavioural interpretations of actions, and the role of internal dispositions. Also important are
the relevance of culture and subculture, behavioural approaches and 'scripts',
and location, products, and services. SCP also concerns offender choice, and
specific offences, opportunity, and intervention. Also considered are SCP
strategies and techniques of crime prevention and how they are evaluated.

Finally, the relevance of SCP to homicide perpetrated by individuals with
severe mental disorder is considered. This covers the predictability of psychotic behaviour, the use of behavioural interventions, and the understanding
of 'internal dispositions' and environmental triggers.

Chapter 4 Demographics and related factors

Using illustrative cases, this chapter considers the mental health of perpetrators of homicide, covering schizophrenia, delusions of persecution, and
psychotic episodes, other disorders, and less specific mental health problems.
Also examined are perpetrator's history of violence, abuse of drugs including
alcohol, refusal to take medication, and distinctions between initial episodes
and patterns of longer-term disorder.

Types of legal outcome of cases are outlined. These are: not guilty because
of insanity, diminished responsibility, mental disease or defect, or not criminally responsible; guilty of manslaughter/second degree murder with diminished responsibility or insanity; and not coming to trial.

Looking firstly at perpetrators, general homicide data gender and age is
presented then considered in relation to cases involving SMD. The chapter
touches on general homicide data on offender's race before considering the

ethnicity and nationality of perpetrators with SMD. Next the chapter looks at the social background/occupation of perpetrators with SMD, whether unemployed, employed, student, or home-based parent. Instances of single and multiple victims are discussed.

Turning to victims, general homicide data on gender and age is briefly examined. Then the age and gender of perpetrators with SMD and their victims is compared. For homicides generally, victims' race is touched on. Next the ethnicity and nationality of perpetrators with SMD and their victims is examined. The social background and occupation of offenders with SMD and their victims is compared. Finally, the chapter discusses relationships between perpetrator and victim in general homicide, and where the perpetrator has SMD. This concerns family members, strangers, friends or acquaintances, and professional relationships.

Part 2 Prevention

Chapter 5 Research into homicide and SMD

This chapter considers research on violence and homicide relating to SMD, focusing particularly on psychotic illness and on research having preventive implications. Firstly, it looks at examples of general risk factors (such as poverty) associated with later violence and their interaction with mental disorder.

Following this, the chapter examines research into homicides perpetrated by individuals with SMD over time and the possible influence of a policy of decreasing the number and capacity of long-stay psychiatric hospitals (deinstitutionalisation). The section after this discusses whether there is an increased risk of homicide associated with SMD. Next, types and aspects of SMD are discussed in relation to violence. These are schizophrenia in general, early and late start offences, delusions (of persecution, misidentification, threat, and control), and hallucinations generating negative emotions and involving commands.

The chapter examines issues concerning procedure, compliance, and behaviour linked to violence risk. These issues relate to better and more focused treatment, not taking prescribed medication, substance abuse, a previous history of violence, and lack of contact with mental health services.

Finally, the difficulties of predicting violence and the role of risk factors in assessment are examined.

Chapter 6 Situational Crime Prevention, homicide, and SMD: Cases

This chapter considers examples of cases between 2015 and 2020 involving perpetrators with SMD. These are Lewis-Ranwell's killing of three elderly men; Christian Lacey's stabbing of his mother after being released from police custody; the decapitation in Russia of a child by her nanny Gyulchekhra Bobokulova; and Timchang Nandap's fatal stabbing of a Dutch engineer in London.

Situational Crime Prevention is used to analyse the four cases, indicating where prevention may have been possible. Equally importantly, the examination shows where preventive techniques which are successful in many other circumstances, are rendered ineffectual. Here alternatives are discussed, sometimes involving pre-emptive action. Reinforcing and supplementing points raised in the chapter, examples are provided of practical situational interventions.

Chapter 7 Means, motive, opportunity, location

Drawing on recent cases of SMD homicide, this chapter discusses means, motive, opportunity, and location. It firstly provides a brief outline of Situational Crime Prevention to which each feature is later related.

Various means of killing are considered – using edge weapons, beating, and bludgeoning, strangulation, using firearms, driving a vehicle, drowning, and employing multiple means. The use of excessive and dramatic violence, and impromptu weapons and those taken to the scene are discussed.

Motive is considered in relation to psychological and behavioural aspects, homicide, and criminal prosecution. Motives relating to SMD are reviewed: voices commanding action, animosity towards the victim or a wider group, conviction that the victim threatens the perpetrator, beliefs antipathetic to the victim, feelings of persecution and threat, a mission to kill, and unclear possibly drug-related motives.

Examples and types of opportunity are considered relating to weapons, victims, undisturbed privacy, and sudden public attack.

Locations that are discussed are the residence shared by perpetrator and victim, the victim's home (or occasionally workplace), the perpetrator's residence, a public street or area, and inside a vehicle.

Chapter 8 Organisational constraints on prevention

Drawing on cases of homicide by perpetrators with SMD, this chapter examines organisational and related issues such as weak communication that can hinder prevention. It first touches on cases where organisational problems of services did not appear to be central.

The chapter then examines two other cases where reports have been published identifying organisational and related problems in services. Philip Simelane's 2012 killing of Christina Edkins led to reports in 2014 and in 2017; and Marc Carter's stabbing of Gino Nelmes in 2012 was followed by a report in 2014. The chapter considers the remit of such reports, and their bearing on reducing homicide risk.

Next a broader view is taken of 16 cases (including those of Simelane and Carter) that raise organisational concerns. Issues emerging include missed indications of accumulating risk of violence, gaps in the liaison and information sharing within and across services, and weaknesses in listening to and questioning the relatives of individuals with SMD. Other points arising are lack of overarching assessments including longitudinal assessments, symptoms of SMD not being recognised, and inadequate physical and procedural precautions for professionals in relation to individuals with SMD. Insufficient suitable treatment is also discussed.

Chapter 9 Retrospect

The chapter briefly summarises what the book has covered, bringing together the issues that have been examined and their preventive implications.

Chapter 10 Glossary: Homicides by those with SMD

Some twenty-five cases (years 2000 to 2020) are listed each with the following information:

Perpetrator = name, age, gender, nationality, race, social background
Victim = name, age, gender, nationality, race, social background
P-V relationship = perpetrator–victim relationship such as 'mother–child' or 'stranger'
Means = weapon or other means involved
Motive = including perpetrator's apparent beliefs and delusions where relevant
Opportunity = including time and date of homicide
Location = place of homicide such as the victim's home or a public place
Preventative strategy = possible foci of prevention
Legal outcome = court judgement on the perpetrator's culpability
Notes = notable further information
References = references for further reading.

Conclusion

Homicides by individuals with SMD can raise public anxiety and concern. Media coverage including that of the popular press shapes accounts to convey the violence and the unexpectedness of some of these homicides. Discussion of these cases and reaction to them can variously arouse worries about evoking prejudice towards people with mental disorders generally, and may raise concerns that the suffering of victim's families and friends are being minimised. The present book attempts to aid understanding of SMD homicides and to consider risk reduction and prevention.

Suggested activities

Begin to familiarise yourself with the cases in the glossary. Select two or three examples and note the structure of the information including the headings of perpetrator and victim and their relationship; means, motive, opportunity, and location; the legal outcome of the case; and possible preventive strategies.

Look further into one of the cases where internet references provide you with further information.

Key texts

Allely, C. (2020) *The Psychology of Extreme Violence*. London, Routledge.

This engaging, up to date text looks in a multidisciplinary way at extreme violence, drawing on contemporary case studies to illustrate the themes. Serial homicide, mass shooting, school shootings, and lone actor terrorism are included as well as guidance for assessing threat and for prevention.

Farrell, M. (2018) *Psychosis under Discussion: How We Talk about Madness*. Abingdon, Routledge.

This book examines ways people talk about psychosis by considering the relationship between language and perceptions of mental disorder. It discusses historical terms, personal accounts, psychiatric terminology, psychoanalysis and later theoretical developments, advocacy, anti-psychiatry, and slang and humour. Chapter 9 on media coverage of homicides by individuals with SMD discusses television drama, movies, and news stories.

References

Allely, C. (2020) *The Psychology of Extreme Violence*. London, Routledge.
Bernstein, E. and Koppel, N. (2008) 'A death in the family' *Wall Street Journal* (16 August 2008) www.wsj.com/articles/SB121883750650245525.
CNN/KLTV (2003) 'Texas woman, member of Assembly of God, says God told her to kill sons' *Internet Archive* (13 May 2003) www.cephas-library.com/assembly_of_god/assembly_of_god_member_killed_her_sons.html.
Crump, C., Sundquist, K., Winkleby, M. A. and Sundquist, J. (2013) 'Mental disorders and vulnerability to homicidal death: Swedish Nationwide Cohort Study' *British Medical Journal* 346: f557. www.bmj.com/content/346/bmj.f557.
Falkenberg, L. (2003) 'Closing arguments begin in Texas mother's murder trial' *Associated Press* (3 April 2003) www.cephas-library.com/assembly_of_god/assembly_of_god_member_killed _her_sons.html.
Farrell, M. (2018) *Psychosis under Discussion: How We Talk about Madness*. Abingdon, Routledge.
Greenwood, C., Brooke, C. and Dolan, A. (2016) *Daily Mail* (17 June 2016, p. 1).
A Hundred Families (2015) *A Practical Guide for Families after a Mental Health Homicide*. www.ahundredfamilies.org.
Linning, S. (2015) 'The real Norman Bates' *Daily Mail On-line* (19 June 2015).
Reed, A. (2014) *Homicide Investigation Report into the Death of a Child* (STEIS reference 2013/7122) www.birminghamandsolihullccg.nhs.uk/about-us/publications/safeguarding/527-christina-edkins-homicide-investigation-report/file.

Reporter (2013) '1,200 killed by mental patients: Shock 10-year toll exposes care crisis' *Sun* (7 October 2013) www.thesun.co.uk/sol/homepage/news/5183994/1200-killed-by-mental-patients-in-shock-10-year-toll.html.

Sontag, D. (2011) 'A schizophrenic, a slain worker, troubling questions' *New York Times* (16 June 2011).

TASS (2016) 'The murder of a child in Moscow: Investigation progress and public reaction' *TASS* (29 February 2016) https://tass.ru/proisshestviya/2706157 (in Russian).

United Nations Office on Drugs and Crime (2013) *Global Study on Homicide*. Vienna, Austria: UNODCwww.unodc.org/documents/data-and-analysis/gsh/Booklet1.pdf.

Part 1

Understanding

Chapter 2

Understanding SMD, homicide, and prevention

Introduction

This chapter considers definitions and types of SMD especially in relation to disorders relevant to homicides described in the book's glossary and discussed in later chapters. As many such disorders involve psychotic features, the chapter describes psychosis and how it is either fundamentally related or associated with SMDs. This involves examining schizophrenia, substance/medication-induced psychotic disorder, depressive disorder, and manic episodes. For each of these, the chapter considers a brief definition, diagnostic criteria, prevalence, risk factors, and treatment.

Turning to a discussion of homicide, the chapter considers how it is categorised, including according to the relationship between perpetrator and victim. Legal understandings of insanity and the tests of criminal responsibility are outlined. Reference is made to cases of homicide perpetrated by individuals with SMD. Prevention is discussed in general and in relation to homicide looking at both longer term approaches and more immediate steps.

Severe mental disorder

Frequently, the expressions, 'severe mental disorder', 'severe mental illness', and 'severe psychiatric disorders' are used interchangeably. SMD refers to people with 'psychological problems that are often so debilitating that their ability to engage in functional and occupational activities is severely impaired' (Public Health England, 2018). A similar definition is of 'a mental, behavioural, or emotional disorder resulting in a serious functional impairment, which substantially interferes with or limits one or more major life activities' (National Institute for Mental Health, February 2019 update). Often referred to as 'severe mental illnesses' are schizophrenia and bipolar disorder (Public Health England, 2018). More broadly, SMD has been taken to include, 'schizophrenia, bipolar disorder, schizoaffective disorder, and major depressive disorder' (De Hert, Correll and Bobes, 2011, p. 52). Highlighting the link with psychosis, Torrey (2012) refers to 'severe psychiatric

DOI: 10.4324/9781003172727-3

disorders' as embracing schizophrenia, bipolar disorder with psychosis, and depression with psychosis (Ibid. p. 5).

Psychosis and its role in disorders

Definition of psychosis and its wide application

Concisely, psychosis is 'a mental disorder characterised by gross impairment in reality testing'. It is indicated by 'delusions, hallucinations, markedly incoherent speech and disorganised or agitated behaviour'. Usually the individual is apparently unaware of the 'incomprehensibility of this behaviour' (Anderson, 2007, p. 1573).

Psychosis is not of itself strictly a mental disorder but refers to the symptoms of some conditions such as schizophrenia which broadly indicate a detachment from reality. Most commonly they include hallucinations (seeing, hearing, and feeling things that are not real to others) and delusions (believing things that are not true). A period of psychosis may be referred to as a 'psychotic episode'. In SMDs psychosis can be either a fundamental or an associated aspect.

Someone may be referred to as 'psychotic' if they have the symptoms indicative of psychosis, especially if a recognisable disorder (such as schizophrenia) is not identified. One can say that someone has psychosis and that they also have for example schizophrenia in the sense that the former refers to symptoms and the latter to a mental disorder.

Key features of psychosis

In the widely used *Diagnostic and Statistical Manual of Mental Disorders Fifth Edition* (hereafter, *DSM-5*) (American Psychiatric Association, 2013), key features of psychosis are identified as:

1   Delusions
2   Hallucinations
3   Disorganised speech
4   Grossly disorganised or catatonic behaviour
5   Negative symptoms (American Psychiatric Association, 2013, p. 99).

Delusions are rigid beliefs that are 'not amenable to change in the light of conflicting evidence' (Ibid. p. 87). Typical delusions are persecutory, referential, grandiose, and 'bizarre'. Delusions of persecution, the most common, involve a belief that the individual is to be harmed or harassed by another person or organisation. (They are sometimes still referred to as delusions of paranoia or more briefly 'paranoia' but this term is increasingly considered rather vague). Other typical delusions are 'referential' ones in which a person believes that certain comments, gestures, or environmental cues are directed at them. With grandiose delusions individuals may incorrectly believe that they are famous, possess great wealth, or have outstanding ability. 'Bizarre' delusions might include those of thought withdrawal, thought insertion, or control. With delusions of thought withdrawal, an outside force is believed to have removed the person's thoughts. Regarding 'thought insertion' people believe that alien thoughts have been put into their mind. With 'delusions of control' it is held that one's body or actions are being operated by an outside force (Ibid.).

Hallucinations are involuntary 'perception-like experiences' but they occur without an external stimulus (Ibid.). In schizophrenia and related conditions, the most usual hallucinations are auditory ones. These are usually voices, which may be familiar or unfamiliar and which are perceived as 'distinct from' the individuals' own thoughts. Hallucinations may be in other sensory modes such as sensations of touch and smell that have the full force of reality (Ibid.).

With disorganised speech the individual may switch from one topic to another or respond to questions in an only partially related or unrelated way. Disorganisation is generally so severe that it substantially impairs communication. Such speech is taken as an indication of disorganised thinking (Ibid., p. 88).

Grossly disorganised or abnormal motor behaviour can include 'unpredictable agitation' and problems in carrying out actions directed at a goal. Catatonic behaviour can refer to a significant decrease in reactions to one's surroundings such as assuming a rigid pose and retaining it for long periods. On the other hand, 'catatonic excitement' which can also occur involves excessive motor activity with no apparent cause (Ibid., p. 88).

'Negative symptoms' include reduced emotional expression such as reflected in facial expression, eye contact, and flat speech. Other negative symptoms are a decline in 'motivated self-initiated purposeful activities', diminished speech output, and a reduced ability to experience pleasure from positive experiences (Ibid., p. 88).

Disorders with which psychosis is fundamental or associated

DSM-5 (American Psychiatric Association, 2013) provides diagnostic criteria for several psychotic disorders grouped as 'Schizophrenia spectrum and other psychotic disorders' in which psychosis is integral (Ibid., pp. 87–122). These include: 'schizophrenia', 'delusional disorder', 'brief psychotic disorder', 'schizophreniform disorder', 'schizoaffective disorder', and 'substance/medication-induced psychotic disorder'. Psychosis is also integral in 'schizotypal personality disorder'.

Other disorders can be 'associated with' psychotic episodes. Psychotic features can be found in major depressive disorder and persistent depressive disorder (American Psychiatric Association, 2013, pp. 155–188) and in bipolar disorder, a feature of which is manic episodes (Ibid., pp. 123–154).

In the sections below the focus is:

- schizophrenia
- substance/medication-induced psychotic disorder
- depressive disorder
- manic episodes

Schizophrenia

Definition

Schizophrenia is defined as, 'a serious mental illness that affects how a person thinks, feels and behaves'. Individuals with schizophrenia may feel as if they, 'have lost touch with reality' (National Institute of Mental Health, May 2020 revision). Kasper and Papadimitriou (2009) stress that, 'Schizophrenia is a disease of the brain' emphasising their view that it is 'a real (physical) disease like diabetes, epilepsy and high blood pressure' (Ibid., xiii).

Challenges in defining schizophrenia (and many other types of SMD) are widely recognised.

As Torrey (2012) points out, its definition 'is a source of continuing debate'. Certainly, there are many 'abnormalities in brain structure and function' that can be associated with schizophrenia, but no single, measurable feature that can confirm the condition. It is also likely that schizophrenia encompasses more than one 'disease entity' (Ibid., p. 59). Given the current state of understanding, it is necessary to define schizophrenia according to its symptoms. This is not ideal as the same symptoms can be caused by different conditions.

Diagnostic criteria

DSM-5 (American Psychiatric Association, 2013) provides diagnostic criteria for schizophrenia. They are listed A through F. For example, specifications for criterion A indicates some key aspects. Two or more of five possible features must be present for a 'significant period of time' during a month (less if the condition is successfully treated). The five features are: delusions, hallucinations, disorganised speech, grossly disorganised or catatonic behaviour, and negative symptoms. These are in fact the features of psychosis generally. At least one of the features must be delusions, hallucinations, or disorganised speech (American Psychiatric Association, 2013, p. 99).

For a 'significant time' from the start of the disturbance, in one or more areas such as work, self-care, or interpersonal relations, the 'level of functioning is … markedly below the level achieved prior to the onset'. If the disorder started in childhood or adolescence, there should be evidence of 'failure to achieve expected levels of interpersonal, academic or occupational functioning' (American Psychiatric Association, 2013, p. 103). Reflecting the challenges of schizophrenia, the guidance states, 'The predictors of course and outcome are largely unexplained, and course and outcome may not be reliably predicted' (American Psychiatric Association, 2013, p. 102).

In discussing schizophrenia, *DSM-5* (American Psychiatric Association, 2013) includes 'risk and prognostic factors', the season of birth, and growing up in an urban environment. Diagnostic issues include 'culture and socio-economic factors'. Guidance also recognises the cultural and societal dimensions of ideas such as 'witchcraft' and 'hearing God's voice' (Ibid., p. 103).

Schizophrenia with delusions of persecution

As mentioned earlier when discussing psychosis, delusions of persecution involve a belief that the individual is to be harmed or harassed by another person or organisation. These are also sometimes still referred to as 'paranoid delusions'. It is noted that 'someone experiencing a paranoid delusion may believe that they are being harassed or persecuted. They may believe that they are being chased, followed, watched, plotted against or poisoned, often by a family member or friend' (NHS, 2019b).

Prior to 2013, 'paranoid schizophrenia' was classified as a type of schizophrenia by the American Psychiatric Association. However, in 2013, guidance changed (in *DSM-5*).

Paranoia or delusions of persecution was classified as a symptom of schizophrenia rather than as a subtype. In retrospect, the subtypes had limited stability as diagnoses, low reliability, and poor validity. The former subtypes were no longer seen as stable conditions and were not helping in diagnosis or treatment. 'Schizophrenia with paranoia' is a term still sometimes used where the individual experiences delusions of persecution.

Prevalence

Wancata, Freidl and Unger (2009) give the estimates for one-year prevalence for schizophrenia as 0.34 (range 0.22–0.50) and a lifetime prevalence of 0.55 (range 0.37–0.80). Their estimates for one-year prevalence for schizophrenia *disorders* is 0.60 (range 0.36–0.91) and lifetime prevalence as 1.45 (range 0.8–2.37). Such figures based on reviews of disorders or a group of disorders are not exact. They are expressed as a range because of subtleties of the different types of prevalence and the varied nature of the studies reviewed.

Risk factors and schizophrenia

Although the precise causes of schizophrenia are not known, research indicates that a combination of physical, genetic, psychological, and environmental factors increase the likelihood of developing the disorder. Some individuals may be prone to schizophrenia, and stressful or emotional events might trigger a psychotic episode (NHS, 2019a).

Several factors appear to increase the likelihood of schizophrenia. It tends to run in families possibly because different combinations of genes increase vulnerability (although such patterns do not guarantee that schizophrenia will develop). Twin studies indicate that the disorder is partly inherited. If an identical twin develops schizophrenia, the other twin (sharing the same genes) has a 1 in 2 chance of also having the disorder even if raised separately. When a non-identical twin develops schizophrenia, the other twin (having a different genetic makeup) has only a 1 in 8 chance of developing the condition. Given that the chance of developing schizophrenia in the general population is about 1 in 100, it appears that genes are one factor but not the only one. Also associated with the risk of schizophrenia are complications before and at the time of birth, such as low birthweight, premature labour, and a lack of oxygen (asphyxia) during birth. It is possible that these factors subtly effect brain development (NHS, 2019a).

Differences in brain structure have been identified in individuals with schizophrenia but not everyone with schizophrenia has these changes and they can occur in people without the disorder. This suggests that such changes play a partial role. Neurotransmitters (chemicals carrying messages between brain cells) may be implicated because drugs that alter the levels of neurotransmitters relieve some of the symptoms. Schizophrenia may be caused by a change in the level of dopamine and serotonin, possibly an imbalance between the two, or because of changes in bodily sensitivity to the neurotransmitters. Schizophrenia in people at risk may be triggered by stressful events such as divorce, job loss, losing one's home, bereavement, a broken relationship or physical, sexual, or emotional abuse (NHS, 2019a).

Although drugs are not a direct cause, their abuse appears to increase the risk of developing schizophrenia or similar disorders. Cannabis, cocaine, lysergic acid diethylamide (LSD), and amphetamines are among the drugs which may trigger symptoms of schizophrenia among susceptible individuals. Using amphetamines or cocaine can lead to psychosis and can cause a relapse in people recovering from an earlier episode. Teenagers and young adults who are regular cannabis users are more likely to develop schizophrenia as adults (NHS, 2019a).

Treatment

Given that the complex causes of schizophrenia are not fully understood, treatment and therapy involve managing its symptoms and enabling an individual to function day to day. Antipsychotic drugs may be prescribed which can reduce the frequency and strength of psychotic symptoms. Usually administered orally as pills or liquid, some of these medications can be given as injections every few weeks. Where such drugs do not lead to improvement, clozapine may be prescribed which requires the individual to have a blood test to detect the possibility of a potentially dangerous side effect. Many people have side effects when starting antipsychotic medication. These include drowsiness and weight gain. Where such side effects persist, some people may stop taking the medication, which can worsen symptoms. Psychosocial interventions may be used, commonly in combination with antipsychotic medication. These psychosocial interventions include cognitive behavioural therapy, training in behavioural skills, and support for employment (National Institute of Mental Health, May 2020 revision, paraphrased).

Coordinated specialty care (CSC) refers to programmes for people with first episode psychosis. These programmes involve a team of health professionals and specialists who deliver a comprehensive package of provision such as psychotherapy, medication management, case management, support for employment and education, and family education and help. The patient and the team work together to make treatment decisions, as far as possible involving family members. Assertive Community Treatment (ACT) is designed for people with schizophrenia at risk of being homeless or being repeatedly hospitalized. It involves a multidisciplinary team who share the case load, and offer direct service provision, frequent patient contact, low patient to staff ratios, and community outreach (National Institute of Mental Health, May 2020 revision, paraphrased).

Substance/medication-induced psychotic disorder

Definition

An essential point in defining a substance/medication induced psychotic disorder is that it involves, 'prominent delusions and/or hallucinations ... that are judged to be due to the physiological effects of a substance/medication' (American Psychiatric Association, 2013, p. 112).

Diagnostic criteria

In the disorder, either delusions or hallucinations (or both) are present. Additionally, there is evidence that these symptoms developed 'during or soon after' intoxication with a substance or withdrawal from it or after 'exposure to' a medication where these can produce delusions or hallucinations. In important areas of functioning such as social or occupational ones, the disturbance causes 'clinically significant distress or impairment'. Notably, hallucinations that the person realises are substance or medication induced are not included in the criteria (American Psychiatric Association, 2013, pp. 110–113).

Prevalence

The prevalence of this disorder is unknown. Of individuals presenting with a first episode of psychosis in different settings, 7–20% are reported to have substance/medication induced psychotic disorder (American Psychiatric Association, 2013, p. 113).

Risk factors

Effectively, the condition central to substance/medication induced psychotic disorder is psychotic disorder itself. Given this, the risk factors are inappropriately taking certain substances/medications. Medications that can cause substance-induced psychotic disorder include anaesthetics, analgesics, antidepressants, and anticonvulsants. Among psychoactive substances that can cause the disorder are alcohol, cannabis, inhalants, amphetamines, and cocaine. Implicated toxins include volatile substances such as fuel or paint.

Treatment

Treatment involves desisting taking the substance, ensuring a calm setting and often, administering an anxiolytic (such as benzodiazepine or an antipsychotic drug). Where psychosis is owing to dopamine stimulating drugs like amphetamine, an antipsychotic drug is effective. Where the substance does not involve the action of dopamine, an anxiolytic may be helpful, or simply observation may be all that is necessary. Also, with drugs like LSD, quiet observation may be all that is required (Tamminga, 2018).

Depression and major depressive disorder

Definition

Depression involves, 'depressed mood and/or near loss of pleasure in activities that were previously enjoyed'. Often it is associated with somatic manifestations such as weight change or disturbed sleep and with cognitive effects like impaired concentration. It may significantly impair ability to function socially and at work, and increases risk of suicide (Corvell, 2020).

Diagnostic criteria

Diagnostic criteria for major depression includes five or more of nine specified symptoms that have been present for the same two-week period and that differ from previous functioning. These include 'depressed mood' and 'markedly diminished interest or pleasure, in activities' most of the time (American Psychiatric Association, 2013, pp. 160–168, paraphrased).

Major depressive disorder can occur with psychotic features involving delusions and/or hallucinations (Ibid., p. 162). With 'mood congruent' psychotic features, the content of all the hallucinations and delusions are 'consistent with' the usual depressive themes. These are 'personal inadequacy, guilt, disease, death, nihilism, or deserved punishment'. In the case of mood incongruent psychotic features, the content of delusions and hallucinations either lacks such content or is a mixture of mood congruent and incongruent themes (Ibid., p. 186).

Risk factors

First degree family members of people with major depressive disorder have a risk of such disorder two to four times higher than that of the general population. High levels of neuroticism appear to make individuals more susceptible to developing depressive episodes 'in response to stressful life events'. Adverse childhood experiences (especially when they are many and various) are risk factors for depressive disorder (American Psychiatric Association, 2013, p. 166).

Depressive disorders can sometimes be brought about by physical conditions such as brain tumour or stroke, or by some drugs including recreational drugs, and certain beta-blockers (drugs which slow down the heart by blocking the action of hormones like adrenaline) (Corvell, 2020).

Prevalence

In the US, the 12-month prevalence in major depressive disorder is approximately 7%. Within the 18- to 29-year-old age groups there is a three times higher prevalence than in the 60 and over age group.

Treatment

Among drugs used to treat depression, selective serotonin re-uptake inhibitors are often tried first. They appear to work by increasing brain levels of the neurotransmitter serotonin which is believed to positively influence mood and emotion (and sleep). Serotonin after carrying a 'message', is normally reabsorbed by nerve cells (re-uptake) and SSRIs inhibit this re-uptake allowing more serotonin to be available to pass further messages between nearby cells. The resulting rise in serotonin levels can improve symptoms of depression. If SSRIs are ineffective, other drugs are prescribed that effect serotonin and/or norepinephrine. Psychotherapy may be used.

Manic episode

A manic episode is not in itself a mental disorder but can be a symptom of conditions including schizoaffective disorder and bipolar disorder. In the context of bipolar I disorder, criteria for a manic episode includes 'a distinct period of abnormally and persistently elevated, expansive, or irritable mood and abnormally and persistently increased goal-directed activity or energy lasting at least 1 week and present most of the day, nearly every day'.

Three or more of seven symptoms are present during the period of mood disturbance and increased energy or activity. These are 'inflated self-esteem or grandiosity', 'decreased need for sleep', 'more talkative than usual or pressure to keep talking', 'flight of ideas or subjective experience that thoughts are racing', 'distractibility', 'increase in goal directed activity … or psychomotor agitation', and 'excessive involvement in activities that have a high potential for painful consequences' (American Psychiatric Association, 2013, p. 124).

Schizoaffective disorder

In schizoaffective disorder (American Psychiatric Association, 2013, pp. 105–110) there is an 'uninterrupted period of illness' in which there is 'major mood episode'. This mood episode may be 'major depressive' or 'manic'. At some time during this period, criterion A for schizophrenia is present. Also, there are, 'delusion or hallucinations for 2 or more weeks in the absence of a major episode (depressive or manic) during the lifetime duration of the illness'. Symptoms meeting the criteria for a 'major mood episode' are present for most of the duration of the 'active and residual portions of the illness' (Ibid., pp. 105–106).

Schizoaffective disorder is not a distinctive disease category. Accordingly, clinicians are advised to consider 'dimensional assessments' of depression and mania for all psychotic disorders which can alert them to 'mood pathology' and the need to treat it where appropriate (Ibid., p. 90).

Bipolar disorder

A distinction is made between bipolar disorder I and II. Bipolar I disorder (American Psychiatric Association, 2013, pp. 123–132) is essentially a modern version of 'the classic manic-depressive disorder or affective psychosis described in the nineteenth century' (Ibid., p. 133). However, neither psychosis nor the 'lifetime experience of a major depressive episode' is a requirement (p. 123). There is provision though for physicians and others to record when bipolar I disorder occurs with 'mood congruent' or 'mood incongruent' psychotic features and with catatonia (p. 127).

Bipolar II disorder (American Psychiatric Association, 2013, pp. 132–139) involves 'the lifetime experience of at least one episode of major depression and at least one hypomanic episode' (Ibid., p. 123). It can be associated with 'mood congruent' or 'mood incongruent' psychotic features and with catatonia (p. 135).

Prevalence of manic disorders

From the mid-1970s to 2000, the rate of mania (variously labelled 'major affective disorder–bipolar disorder' and 'bipolar I disorder') was stable. It was consistently identified in US and international studies as ranging from 0.4% to 1.6%. Some researchers in the late 1990s to the 2000s reported prevalence for bipolar disorders (I and II and others) as 5% to 7% or more which has been questioned (Yutzy, Woofter, Abbott, Melhem and Parish, 2012).

Risk factors for manic episodes

Risk factors for manic episodes relate to those for the disorders that are associated with them. For example, within the context of bipolar disorder there is evidence that 'mania' may occur when bodily levels of the neuro-transmitter noradrenaline are too high. (Neurotransmitters are chemicals controlling certain brain functions.)

Treatment for manic episodes

Among medication used to treat acute manic episodes are antipsychotics and mood stabilisers. Antipsychotics can reduce symptoms quickly. However, mood stabilisers used long term can help prevent future episodes. Antipsychotics include olanzapine, risperidone, and quetiapine. Among mood stabilisers are lithium, carbamazepine, and divalproex sodium.

Homicide: Legal definitions

At its most basic, homicide involves, 'the death of an individual through the actions of one or more other individuals' (Corzine, 2011, editorial). Among legal definitions of homicide in many countries, certain aspects are common, and law in England and Wales illustrates these core elements. Homicide covers the offences of both murder and manslaughter as well as other cases of a person causing or being involved in the death of another. In such instances bound together under the umbrella term, 'homicide', the general criminal conduct ('actus reus') is the same, that of killing another person.

However, causation differs in different circumstances (Croner, 2008, p. 37). Under common law an offence of murder is committed when 'a person unlawfully kills another human being under the Queen's Peace, with malice aforethought' (Ibid.). For an individual over 18 years, a conviction for murder carries a mandatory sentence of life imprisonment. 'Unlawful killing' includes not only actively causing another's death, but also failing to act after creating a dangerous situation. It can involve acts of commission and omission. Where there is 'malice aforethought' there is an intention to kill or to cause 'grievous bodily harm' (Ibid., p. 38).

Certain 'special defences' allow for a conviction of manslaughter rather than murder, namely, diminished responsibility (impaired mental responsibility); pro-vocation; and a suicide pact (Croner, 2008, p. 39). Where such special defences have led the court to a judgement of manslaughter this is classed as 'voluntary manslaughter'. It may be shown that a defendant caused the death of another person but not that he or she had the required 'mens rea' for murder. In this case, the crime is 'involuntary manslaughter' which can involve a defendant killing another person by, 'an unlawful act which was likely to cause bodily harm; or by gross negligence' (Ibid., p. 41).

Where a person with SMD commits homicide, the crime may be judged to be manslaughter rather than murder because of 'diminished responsibility'. Also, a defendant may be found to be 'not guilty by reason of insanity'.

Types of homicide

Types of homicide are diverse, reflecting different causes, relationships between perpetrator and victim, social context, and motive. Such features of typology can be informative when looking at the prevalence of different types, and at their possible prevention.

Some terms convey perpetrator–victim relationships. Matricide involves killing one's mother while patricide refers to killing one's father. The glossary of the present book outlines cases of sons killing their mothers as with Christian Lacey, Mark Tyler, William Bruce, and Nathan Jones. For example, in the UK, Christian Lacey attacked his father and his half-brother although not fatally and later killed his mother with a knife (Docking, 2018). In 2002, in Swindon, UK, Timothy Crook who had been diagnosed with schizophrenia killed both his parents then drove the bodies 150 miles away where he deposited them in the overgrown land of a house he owned (BBC News, 2015).

Prolicide is a broad term referring to a parent killing their offspring. It can include filicide (the killing of one's child), infanticide (killing one's infant aged 0 to 12 months), and feticide (an act which deliberately kills a foetus). Cases implicating SMD include those of Riana Thaiday, Dena Schlosser, Lisa Diaz, and Deana Laney. In Australia, Riana Thaiday killed her children – three sons, four daughters, and a niece all aged between 2 and 14 years old (Australian Associated Press, 2017). In an instance of infanticide Dena Schlosser amputated the arms of her 11-month-old daughter (Joyner, 2004).

Spouse killing is sometimes designated as uxoricide (where a husband kills his wife) and mariticide (in which a wife kills a husband). No examples of spouse killing were in the cases examined in the present book although in the UK, Percy Wright, considered by his physician to be 'anxious and paranoid' killed his former partner Colette Lynch (Twomey, 2009).

Amicide refers to the killing of a friend. Michael Harris who had schizophrenia killed his long-term friend Carl James on the doorstep of the victim's home (Reporter, 2007).

Another classification of homicide includes reference to the sequence of killings, as with murder–suicide. Mark Tyler shot his mother at her home then days later killed himself with the same gun (BBC, 2013). Types of homicide can be designated according to the perpetrators as when we speak of 'male perpetrated homicide'. Circumstances and location can be designated by terms such as 'domestic homicide'. Mode of killing may be indicated as with 'manual strangulation', 'bludgeoning', 'shooting', or 'stabbing'. Combinations of elements can be conveyed as with 'gangland shooting' which identifies perpetrators and possible victims as well as the means of killing.

As will be seen in a later chapter considering demographics, homicide can be analysed in terms of characteristics of the perpetrator and the victim. Gender, age, race/ethnicity, and social background/occupation of both perpetrator and victim can be informative. Homicide may be male on male, or male on female, female on male, or female on female, each raising different questions and issues. Relationships between the ages of the perpetrator and victim may be important. Their relative social background and occupation may raise questions. Whether the perpetrator and victim are of the same or different ethnic background may be revealing. More specifically, the relationship between a perpetrator and victim may tell a story. Were they strangers? Members of the same family? Lifelong friends? Work colleagues? Lovers?

Legal outcome of homicide cases

Verdicts in the cases where the perpetrator has SMD can include being not guilty because of insanity, diminished responsibility, mental disease, or defect, or being not criminally responsible. They can also include instances where the verdict was manslaughter/second degree murder with diminished responsibility and insanity.

In criminal courts, 'insanity' is not a psychiatric condition but a legal term. If an offender is charged with murder, a defence of 'not guilty by reason of insanity' (NGRI) may be made. As Hickey (2008) points out, courts often determine the state of mind of the accused before the trial. During trial, a court must determine whether the accused was insane at the time of the killing and to what degree he or she can be held responsible. 'Insanity' as a legal term refers to the state of mind of the accused at the time of the crime, and the accused has only to be deemed insane at that time and not necessarily before or after it. Many jurisdictions place an offender who has claimed to be NGRI in a psychiatric facility irrespective of their current state of mind (Ibid., p. 59 paraphrased).

In the United States, the Supreme Court ruled that insanity could continue after the criminal act and that an individual found not guilty by reason of insanity of a misdemeanour crime could be involuntarily placed in a psychiatric facility until no longer a danger to themselves or others (*Jones v The United States* (1983)).

Legal determination of insanity

Legal determination of insanity usually relates to tests of criminal responsibility. Formulated in the nineteenth century, the McNaghton Rule (sometimes rendered as the M'Naghton Rule) rests on a relatively simple definition. To demonstrate a defence of insanity it must be proved that at the time of the committing of the act the party accused was labouring under such a defect of reason from disease of the mind as not to know the nature and quality of the act he was doing; or, if he did know, that he did not know he was doing what was wrong. (McNaghten's Case (1843–1860))

Critics consider that McNaghten does not encompass situations in which offenders can distinguish right and wrong but cannot control their behaviour. An additional 'Irresistible Impulse Test' can be used to help determine that the offender, although recognising the difference between right and wrong, was unable to control themselves while committing the offence.

The Brawner Rule effectively combines the intentions of the McNaghten Rule and the Irresistible Impulse Test. It states,

> A person is not responsible for criminal conduct if at the time of such conduct as a result of mental disease or defect he lacks substantial capacity either to appreciate the criminality (wrongfulness) of his conduct or to conform his conduct to the requirement of the law.
>
> (*United States v Brawner*, 1972)

Notice that 'lack of substantial capacity' does not require that there is total impairment.

Some defendants are considered incompetent to stand trial. This does not relate to a court's determination of criminal responsibility because, not standing trial, they are not guilty of any criminal offence. Also, the defendant's state of mind when committing the criminal act may differ from his state of mind when coming to court. Someone found incompetent to stand trial is likely to be placed in a psychiatric setting until medical specialists consider that they are competent, at which time they must stand trial.

Severe mental disorders and homicide cases

It is often pointed out that homicide committed by perpetrators with SMD is comparatively rare, and this is so. It is also worth noting that the impact of such killings can be wide. The homicides are sometimes multiple. Riana Thaiday killed her six children and a niece, Alexander Lewis-Randall bludgeoned to death three elderly men, Timothy Crook killed both his parents, Gregory Davies stabbed to death a mother and son, Deana Laney killed two of her children, and David Attias ran over four pedestrians. Whether one or several victims are killed, the effect spreads grief and fear to family, friends, and the wider community, especially where the killing is dramatically violent.

This section briefly revisits the disorders already outlined and touches on cases where the disorders arise. Reports of homicide have mentioned specific disorders or symptoms which may overlap. Consequently, in some instances more than one type or aspect of SMD was identified as with Timchang Nandap who had schizophrenia, delusions of persecution, and psychosis including hallucinations (Baker, 2018).

Commonly found and sometimes overlapping aspects of SMD were schizophrenia (Alexander Lewis-Ranwell, Gyulchekhra Bobokulova, Philip Simelane, Marc Carter, Michael Harris, Timothy Crook, Davidov, Ronald Dixon, William Bruce, Peter Atkins); delusions of persecution (Alexander Lewis-Ranwell, Alexander Bonds, Timchang Nandap, Philip Simelane, Marc Carter, Timothy Crook, William Bruce, Percy Wright); and psychosis including hallucinations (Christian Lacey, Timchang Nandap, Deyan Devanov, Deana Laney, Riana Thaiday, Ronald Dixon, Dena Schlosser, Marie West).

Occasionally identified were depression (Dena Schloser, Gregory Davis) and mania (Ronald Dixon), obsessive fear and psychosomatic disorders (Lisa Diaz), social anxiety (Gregory Davis), and odd beliefs not necessarily indicating SMD (Deana Laney). Sometimes there were general mental health concerns although a specific condition may not have been identified (David Attias, Keith Addy, Nathan Jones, and Mark Tyler).

Also relating to SMD and increased risk of violence/homicide is the coexistence of other factors sometimes referred to as comorbidity. For example, the coexistence of substance abuse or personality disorder, along with other SMDs that have been discussed, can contribute to increased risk of homicide.

Prevention and related issues

Prevention as involving immediate and longer-term action

'Prevention' refers to an action to prevent something arising, or to stop it happening. The distinction between 'arising' and 'happening' hinges on the time involved, the idea 'arising' suggesting a long continuation and 'happening' implying a sudden occurrence. With homicide as with prevention in general, the aim is to prevent it 'arising', or to stop it 'happening', implying respectively a longer process or a more immediate intervention.

Addressing the events preceding a homicide may involve pre-emptively taking steps over a long period such as enforcing gun control, improving the security of possible targets, and increasing police presence in potential hot spots such as places where criminals congregate. Where there is reason to suspect that a homicide may take place, such as where threats have been made, steps may be taken over a sustained period to prevent this, such as imposing legal restrictions on the movements of the potential perpetrator, protecting the possible victim, and setting up an alarm system for the victim to alert police.

Stopping a homicide at, or close to, its final point can involve urgent steps at the last moment after an attack has occurred to save the life of the victim.

Petherick and Petherick (2019) draw attention to the importance of emergency medical care in this respect. Although such care is not 'a way of preventing homicide as such', it does influence homicide rates. If someone is injured but not immediately killed, the response rates and the lifesaving procedures that are used will affect how many victims survive the incident (Ibid., pp. 305–306).

Reducing homicide

Not all homicides can be prevented, indeed perhaps the majority cannot, so that it may be more accurate to speak not of prevention but of reduction. Among factors that can reduce homicides are, 'the role of the police, public education campaigns, the importance of warning signs, gun control, and emergency medical care' (Petherick and Petherick, 2019, p. 306).

Conclusion

Underpinning many SMDs is psychosis characterised by delusions, hallucinations, disorganised speech, grossly disorganised or catatonic behaviour, and negative symptoms.

Among SMDs are disorders or aspects of disorders including schizophrenia (sometimes with delusions of persecution), substance/medication-induced psychotic disorder, depressive disorder, and manic episodes.

Schizophrenia is a serious mental disorder affecting how a person thinks, feels, and behaves and is associated with losing touch with reality. It can involve delusions of persecution in which the individual believes that they are being harmed or harassed by another person or organisation.

Substance/medication induced psychotic disorder involves prominent delusions and/or hallucinations owing to the physiological effects of a substance or medication. Psychoactive substances that can cause this disorder include alcohol, cannabis, inhalants, amphetamines, and cocaine while among implicated medications are anaesthetics, analgesics, antidepressants, and anticonvulsants.

Depression involves depressed mood and/or great or total diminution of pleasure in activities previously enjoyed. It may be associated with weight change, disturbed sleep, and poor concentration, and can significantly impair ability to function at work and socially, and increases suicide risk.

A manic episode is not in itself a mental disorder but can be a symptom of other disorders including schizoaffective disorder and bipolar disorder. It involves expansive, or irritable mood and 'goal-directed activity or energy' that are abnormally and persistently increased. Symptoms can include an inflated sense of self-esteem or grandiosity, less need for sleep, being more talkative than usual, 'flight of ideas', or racing thoughts, distractibility, higher goal directed activity or mental and physical agitation, and excessive involvement in activities having likely painful consequences.

Homicide involves killing another person with varying degrees of culpability reflected in different terms including 'degrees' of murder, and manslaughter. In legal proceedings, special defences allow a conviction less than murder and include 'diminished responsibility' (impaired mental responsibility). Typologies of homicide often reflect the relationship between perpetrator and victim as with 'matricide'. Means of killing may be indicated such as 'strangling'. Other categorisations include 'murder–suicide', and 'domestic homicide'.

Where a person with SMD commits homicide, they may be judged to have committed manslaughter rather than murder because of 'diminished responsibility'. Also, a defendant may be found to be 'not guilty by reason of insanity' or 'not criminally responsible'. Legal determination of insanity usually relates to tests of criminal responsibility, for example, the McNaghton Rule.

In preventing homicide, the aim is to avoid homicide 'arising', or to stop it 'happening', implying respectively a longer process or a more immediate intervention. As many homicides are not preventable, it may be more realistic to speak of reducing homicides.

Suggested activities

Select a case from the glossary and review the type of SMD that was indicated, the characteristics of the homicide, the legal outcome, and the possible strategies for prevention.

Next, identify and consider at least one case for each of the types of SMD that have been discussed (schizophrenia, delusions of persecution, psychosis including hallucinations, mania, depression, and general mental health concerns).

Key texts

American Psychiatric Association (2013) *Diagnostic and Statistical Manual of Mental Disorders Fifth Edition*. Washington DC, APA.

This manual is a very widely used psychiatric diagnostic guide.

Hough, R. M. and McCorkle, K. D. (2019) (2nd edition) *American Homicide*. Thousand Oaks, CA and London, Sage.

This well-structured book covers homicide data and theories, types of homicide, and court procedures. Although concentrating on American homicide, the text compares this with trends worldwide.

Petherick, W. and Petherick, N. (2019) *Homicide*. San Diego, CA, Elsevier Academic Press.

This book examines homicide with an international perspective focusing on major western nations. It looks at incidence prevalence; the roots of homicide such as biological, psychological, and sociological; types of homicide; investigation and prevention.

References

American Psychiatric Association (2013) *Diagnostic and Statistical Manual of Mental Disorders, Fifth Edition*. Washington DC, APA.

Anderson, D. M. (Chief Lexicographer) (2007) *Dorland's Illustrated Medical Dictionary* (31st edition). Philadelphia, PA, Saunders, Elsevier.

Australian Associated Press (2017) 'Mother psychotic when she killed eight children, Queensland court rules' *Guardian* (4 May 2017) www.theguardian.com/australia-news/2017/may/ 04/mother-psychotic-when-she-killed-eight-children-queensland-court-rules.

Baker, K. (2018) 'Why was mentally ill man set free to kill my husband?' *Mail Online* (2 July 2018) www.dailymail.co.uk/news/article-5909435/Psychotic-killer-stabbed-renowned-academic-death-outside-home.html.

BBC (2013) 'Mental health review after Cray's Hill double death incident' BBC News (27 March 2013) www.bbc.co.uk/news/uk-england-essex-21951670.

BBC News (2015) 'Manslaughter: Timothy Crook guilty of killing parents' BBC News (20 July 2015) www.bbc.co.uk/news/uk-england-wiltshire-33599525.

Corvell, W. (2020) 'Depressive Disorders' *MSD Manual* (March 2020) www.msdmanuals.com/en-gb/professional/psychiatric-disorders/mood-disorders/depressive-disorders.

Corzine, J. (2011) 'Theories of homicide' *Homicide Studies* 15, 4, 315–318.

Croner, P. (2008) *Blackstone's Police Manual 2009 – Volume 1 – Crime* (11th edition). Oxford and New York, Oxford University Press.

De Hert, M., Correll, C. U., Bobes, J., Cetkovich-Bakmas, M., Cohen, D., Asai, I., Detraux, J., Gautam, S., Moeller, H-J., Ndetei, D. M., Newcomer, J. W., Uwakwe, R. and Leucht, S. (2011) 'Physical illness in patients with severe mental disorders. I: Prevalence, impact of medications and disparities in health care' *World Psychiatry* 10, 1, 52–77.

Docking, N. (2018) 'Man stabbed his mum to death and tried to kill his gran's carer in psychotic episode' *Echo* (21 December 2018) www.liverpoolecho.co.uk/ news/liverpool-news/christian-lacey-liz-lacey-murder-15584632.

Hickey, E. W. (2008) *Serial Murderers and Their Victims* (5th edition). Belmont CA, Wadsworth.

Jones v The United States (1983) 463 U.S. 354 (1983).

Joyner, J. (2004) 'Mom cut off baby's arms' *Outside the Beltway* (23 November 2004) www.outsidethebeltway.com/mom_cut_off_babys_arms/.

Kasper, S. and Papadimitriou, G. N. (Eds) (2009) *Schizophrenia: Biopsychosocial Approaches and Current Challenges* (2nd edition) (Medical Psychiatry Series). New York and London, Informa Healthcare.

McNaghten's Case [1843–1860] All ER Rep 229 at 233–234; (1843) 8 ER 718.

National Institute for Mental Health (February 2019 update) 'Mental Illness' www.nimh.nih.gov/health/statistics/mental-illness.shtml.

National Institute of Mental Health (May 2020 revision) 'Schizophrenia' www.nimh.nih.gov/health/topics/schizophrenia/index.shtml.

NHS (11 November 2019a) 'Schizophrenia – causes' www.nhs.uk/conditions/schizophrenia/causes/.

NHS (11 November 2019b) 'Schizophrenia – symptoms' www.nhs.uk/conditions/ schizophrenia/symptoms/.

Public Health England (2018) 'Severe mental illness (SMI) and physical health inequalities' Public Health England (27 September 2018) www.gov.uk/government/publications/

severe-mental-illness-smi-physical-health-inequalities/severe-mental-illness-and-physical-health-inequalities-briefing.

Reporter (2007) 'Schizophrenic addicted to skunk cannabis killed best friend' *Evening Standard* (2 August 2007) www.standard.co.uk/news/schizophrenic-addicted-to-skunk-cannabis-killed-best-friend-6602755.html.

Torrey, E. F. (2012) *The Insanity Offence: How America's Failure to Treat the Seriously Mentally Ill Endangers Its Citizens.* New York and London, W. W. Norton.

Twomey, J. (2009) 'Fury after psychotic killer walks free after four years' *Express* (22 April 2002) www.express.co.uk/news/uk/96406/Fury-as-psychotic-killer-walks-free-after-4-years

United States v Brawner (1972) 471 F. 2d 969 (D. C. Cir. 1972).

Tamminga, C. (2018) 'Substance/medication-induced psychotic disorder' *MSD Manual* (October 2018) www.msdmanuals.com/en-gb/professional/psychiatric-disorders/schizophrenia-and-related-disorders/substance-medication%E2%80%93induced-psychotic-disorder.

Wancata, J., Freidl, M. and Unger, A. (2009). 'Epidemiology and gender' in Kasper, S. and Papadimitriou, G. (Eds) *Schizophrenia: Biopsychosocial Approaches and Current Challenges* (2nd edition). London, Informa Healthcare (pp. 16–25).

Yutzy, S. H., Woofter, C. R., Abbott, C. C., Melhem, I. M. and Parish, B. S. (2012) 'The increasing frequency of mania and bipolar disorder causes and potential negative impacts' *Journal of Nervous Mental Disorders* 200, 5, 380–387.

Chapter 3

Understanding Situational Crime Prevention

Introduction

Situational Crime Prevention (SCP) is introduced focusing on its effectiveness, development, aspects and features, strategies and techniques, and its application to homicide by perpetrators with severe mental disorder. The development of SCP is described from its origins in the study of boys absconding from a boarding school for 'delinquents'.

Features of SCP include the theoretical underpinnings of the approach and how these lead to strategies for prevention; related theories; and the behavioural interpretations of actions and the role of internal dispositions. Other aspects are the relevance of culture and subculture; behavioural approaches and 'scripts'; and location, products and services. Also important are offender choice; and specific offences, opportunity, and intervention. Each of these is explained.

The chapter considers SCP strategies and techniques of crime prevention and how they are evaluated. Finally, the relevance of SCP to homicide perpetrated by individuals with severe mental disorder is considered. This involves looking at the predictability of psychotic behaviour, behavioural interventions, and understanding 'internal dispositions' and environmental triggers.

Situational Crime Prevention and Its Effectiveness

Situational Crime Prevention (SCP) is an approach to crime reduction involving strategies and techniques originally developed from the work of UK researcher Ron Clarke (Clarke, 1967). The approach has a record of successful interventions in many areas in which it has been applied. For example, a 'secure by design' strategy which draws on SCP involves encouraging good practice in urban planning so that crime prevention is considered in the design stage of proposals. This includes minimum standards of physical security, a minimum number of access points, maximum natural surveillance, good management and maintenance policies, and a mix of dwellings to exert informal control. An evaluation of 25 secure by design and non-secure by design housing estates indicated that in the former total crime fell by 55% (Armitage, 2000).

DOI: 10.4324/9781003172727-4

Arizona State University Center for Problem Oriented Policing (various dates) publishes problem-specific guides covering a wide range of issues and evidence for their working. They include a guide relating to people with mental disorders as offenders and as victims (Cordner, 2006).

SCP does not limit its view of reducing crime only to the work of police, probation services, the courts, and prisons but spreads its remit much wider than the criminal justice system. Aiming to reduce opportunities for offending, SCP first analyses the circumstances that engender specific kinds of crime, recognising that there are in certain situations and settings opportunities to commit offences. It then uses modifications to the environment and to the management of situations to change how opportunity is structured for those crimes to take place (Clarke, 2018, abstract). This will become clearer as fuller descriptions and examples of SCP are provided later. But before this, it is necessary to examine the theories that lie behind the practical strategies and techniques.

Origins and development of SCP

What does SCP seek to do and how does it set about doing it? Essentially, SCP aims to reduce opportunities for offending using the steps of analysing and modifying to change the way that opportunities for crime arise. SCP analyses the circumstances which lead to specific kinds of crime. Then, it seeks to modify the environment and the behaviour of those involved. These modifications are made to change the way that opportunities for crime are presented or perceived for those crimes to take place. In the terminology of SCP, the approach makes 'managerial and environmental modifications' to change the 'opportunity structure' for crime (Clarke, 2018, abstract).

As a situational approach, SCP scrutinises specific types of crimes. It identifies aspects of the situation in which the behaviour occurs that encourages or aids the transgression. The situation is assumed (at least in part) to influence the choice and intention to commit a crime. It follows that altering or removing factors that make up the situation will reduce opportunities for the crime to be perpetrated. Although the situation is the focus, SCP does not dismiss the possible motivation of the perpetrator. However, it does propose that the motivation to carry out a specific type of crime is influenced by the situation and the cues associated with it. A potential offender's intention to transgress reduces where such cues are removed. Preventive measures are therefore viewed as constraining.

The way that SCP was initiated and developed also illustrates how it is tied to specific situations, how they are analysed, and how the environment is modified to reduce opportunities for offending. Ron Clarke who originated SCP was a research officer at the Kingswood Training School, Bristol, England. Kingswood was then a boarding school for delinquent boys. A challenge facing the establishment was the number of boys running away ('absconding'). Rather than focus solely on the possible reasons or motivations for boys absconding, Clarke examined the situations in which these events occurred.

Analysing the records of these incidents, he noticed that certain features offered opportunities for the boys to run away from the school.

For example, when the nights grew longer towards winter, absconding was higher than in summer when nights were shorter. Winter nights provided more time for boys to get away under cover of darkness when staff were less likely to notice. In other words, the 'opportunity structure' included seasons of the year and staff awareness (Clarke, 1967). Modifications to change this opportunity structure (that is reducing the opportunities) might be to ensure that the areas round the school were better lit, and to increase staffing levels and staff vigilance during seasons when nights were long. This would be expected to prevent offending behaviour. More generally, if situations provide an opportunity structure, it might be possible to develop interventions that reduce such opportunities. This would constrain chances to offend, in line with SCP (Clarke, 1980).

Accordingly, researchers working with police and others who see the potential of SCP have focused on specific problems and situations. As these have been analysed and modifications to the situation have been identified, a wide range of police strategies has developed (Arizona State University Center for Problem Oriented Policing, various dates). These are sometimes referred to as problem-oriented strategies because they identify a problem situation, analyse it, and seek to modify aspects which provide opportunities for a specific crime. Various features of SCP contribute to how this problem orientated approach works.

Features of SCP

Preventive aspects of theories of crime

Several well-known theories explain aspects of crime but fall short in proposals for preventing it. Kohlberg's (1978) theory of moral development suggests that long term re-education in moral reasoning might be beneficial. Control theory (Hirschi, 1969) points to broad re-education involving social, psychological, and moral elements to ensure that rules are followed. Labelling theory (Becker, 1963) challenges tendencies in the legal system and in society that constrain an offender to a single negative identity and involve a process of 'secondary deviance'. Its implications are that if negative labelling is avoided, repeated criminal acts would be reduced. Strain theory (Merton, 1938) and its adaptations (Agnew, 2001) suggests that crime might be reduced by making fundamental changes to social structure and to the way status in society is signalled. Such theories imply variously very long-term approaches to changing individuals through re-education and training, or deep changes in society, social structure, legal systems, and social status. In short, they tend to offer long-term, diffuse approaches rather than direct, shorter term problem focused strategies.

By contrast, differential reinforcement theory and rational choice theory which underpin SCP point to strategies for prevention. In examining the theoretical background to SCP, we will see the contributions made by behavioural perspectives and by the exercise of rational choice. In subsequent sections of this chapter concerning SCP, I am indebted to the framework provided by Freilich and Newman (2019).

Theories and SCP strategies

Many SCP techniques relate to theories which imply that a perpetrator of crime has certain tendencies and acts in particular ways. Furthermore, individuals are taken to behave rationally and to make rational choices. They can act independently, that is they exercise 'agency', and behave hedonistically in tending to avoid pain and to seek pleasure. Such a view of rational choice, agency, and hedonism is woven into SCP strategies.

In using some strategies, it is recognised as effective to warn individuals of the consequences of offending, as well as the relative certainty and speed of being apprehended. An example is the use of CCTV cameras providing records of offences leading to speedy action to catch the perpetrator (Cozens, 2008). Other approaches recognise that implementing legally driven punishment takes too long. Consequently, the prospect of distant legal sanctions tends not to influence how offenders make decisions about their criminal activity (Braga and Kennedy, 2012).

It is a well-established precept of behavioural interventions that punishment can effectively shape behaviour if it immediately follows unwanted behaviour. Applied to crime, punishment can deter if it directly follows the offence, suggesting that delayed consequences are ineffective. Accordingly, SCP is sceptical about long delayed formal punishment and prefers instead prompt, or constantly present, situational interventions.

Some interventions hinder crime being committed, like controlling the exits and entrances to stores so that anyone stealing items must evade security and surveillance hurdles. This assumes that a potential offender will choose to conform because the increased 'costs' make it less worthwhile to offend.

SCP recognises the role of publicity in reducing crime. Publicizing SCP interventions educates members of the community to take specific informed precautions or preventive actions. For example, authorities in a local area may publicise the importance of a driver locking the car when leaving it in a car park. Vehicle owners may be advised to fit disabling devices to make stealing harder, and more time consuming, and therefore riskier for the thief. Such approaches increase the 'costs' of a perpetrator offending by increasing the risk that they will be apprehended (Bowers and Johnson, 2005). Where an offender is aware of publicity around crime prevention, it can affect their perceptions of the (increased) difficulty and risks of committing a crime and the (higher) chances of being caught.

Behaviourist interpretations of actions and the role of internal dispositions

Some SCP strategies make it impossible for would-be perpetrators to offend, irrespective of their seeming motivation, thought patterns, or emotions

(Cornish and Clarke, 2008, p. 41). 'Hardening targets' can involve setting up physical and personnel security barriers to protect private property. These can be made so robust that they are effectively impassable. Such an approach does not depend on assumptions about the psychology of offenders, the presence of agency, rational choice, or a hedonistic nature. It just stops potential offenders entering the protected site. The individual is expected to respond to a given stimulus predictably, regardless of any supposed internal states or thought processes (Newman and Freilich, 2012, p. 216).

Some 'soft' SCP approaches to reducing crime do not rely upon offender rationality or agency (involving conscious decision making). They rather hypothesise that an offender has internal dispositions towards behaviours that can be provoked by certain characteristics of the environment. These dispositions may lie dormant in the absence of certain situational conditions triggering the related behaviours. In general terms it may be believed that seeing weapons being carried, even by security guards or police officers, suggests that violence is ubiquitous and therefore everyone should be ready to use force. A more behavioural attempt to describe such notions can be made that suggest preventive steps. A police officer who publicly and openly carries weapons can seemingly provoke internal dispositions in some individuals which precipitate their violence. If the stimuli did not arise, the person would not be disposed to offend. Consequently, techniques can be developed to remove environmental cues that trigger offending, suggesting that in some circumstances, police officers conceal their weapons (Wortley, 2008).

SCP in relation to culture and subculture

Researchers using SCP tend to view the concept of social class as too vague and broad to be practically useful in prevention. They prefer to concentrate on specific, concrete situations. Some prevention work in neglected neighbourhoods has drawn effectively on SCP rather than social class interpretations (Freilich and Newman, 2016; Garland, 2000; Wilson and Kelling, 1982). However, while broad notions of social class are treated with caution, culture and subculture have a role.

Subculture may be relevant in certain types of organized crime. Criminals have values and codes of conduct leading to firm beliefs. Brought to the crime situation, these beliefs constitute part of the circumstances that are assessed by those aiming to reduce crime. However, in applying SCP preventive techniques to specified circumstances, authorities need not be overly concerned whether a value is culturally based so long as key features exist. These are that the values and beliefs are empirically identifiable, and that they can be manipulated to modify decision making in a specific situation. For example, with perpetrators, such as American far-right activists, holding extremist beliefs, researchers have used responses shaped by the specified circumstances to prevent offending (Freilich and Chermak, 2009). Drawing on guilt and shame, these techniques are designed to intervene in an individual's decision making at the right time (Wortley, 1996).

Behavioural approaches and scripts

An important feature of SCP is an understanding of 'scripts'. Just as an actor's script sets out the content and structure of a role, so the understanding of behavioural scripts offers a sequence of expected behaviours. This includes for a specified situation the typical roles that are involved, the setting, the items in the setting, and the expected sequence of events. In shopping, typical roles are the storekeeper and the customer. The setting is the store. Items might be groceries or hardware or whatever the shop specialises in as well as a cash register and a counter. An expected sequence of events would be that a customer enters the store, selects several items, pays for them, puts them in a bag, and departs. This provides a framework for what to expect when you enter a store. Variations will arise according to the size of the store, whether it is self-service and so on, but the script forms a framework for what to expect.

Applied to criminal behaviour, scripts concern the situation in which a crime occurs. Among relevant roles are likely to be those of the criminal, victim, and witnesses. Different settings may be a house being burgled, a public place where a victim is attacked, or a store being robbed. Items involved may be burglary tools, offensive weapons, or computers used for hacking. In a burglary, the sequence of events may be reconnoitring a property before the crime takes place, later approaching the property unseen, entering it undetected, finding valuables, gathering them to be taken away, and escaping unnoticed with the goods. Each of these steps can be broken down further. Finding the valuables for example may involve a systematic search of a property. Alternatively, previous intelligence may have been gathered, enabling the burglar to go directly to the section of the property where valuables are kept. In each part of the sequence the offender makes decisions and acts in response to the situation, as when an owner unexpectedly returns to a property, or a burglar alarm is seen attached to the building.

SCP using a script approach analyses the decisions and actions that an offender follows in carrying out the crime. This forms a 'procedural analysis' (Cornish, 1994). There are overall goals and sub-goals involved in committing a crime. In a violent attack the sub-goals may include obtaining a weapon, ensuring that the proposed victim is alone or unguarded, and escaping after the attack. In crime scripts, there are sequences of decisions and actions associated with reaching such sub-goals. Obtaining a weapon may involve making it, stealing it or purchasing it. These sub-goals contribute towards the overall goals of the crime (Cornish and Clarke, 2002, p. 47).

Location, products, and services

Given that the setting of an offence is part of the script of a crime, scripts are relevant when considering the location of an offence. Analysing the geography of crimes emerges from this. Patterns of criminal events and activities relate to places such as street corners and neighbourhoods and are associated with certain times (Brantingham and Brantingham, 1981). Police or private security personnel may be able to use such information to concentrate a presence in these settings and to intervene to stop the offence.

Design of products and services can make it more difficult for a would-be offender to carry out a crime (Ekblom, 2012a, 2012b). A vehicle may have extra security features such as a concealed switch to disconnect the engine from controls, extra thick glass windows, and alarms. Or a vehicle used by a potential victim such as a police officer may have bullet proof windows.

Offender choice

SCP approaches imply that an offender's actions are not random and irrational. This suggests predictability in the choices or decisions that offenders make and the actions that they take. However, context is also important. Offenders will have certain perceptions of their needs (and goals) based to a greater or lesser degree on reason. Criminals will also have perceptions of the opportunities presented by the environment that will enable or interfere with their actions. Both perceptions of personal needs and environmental opportunities contribute to how the person behaves in the situation.

With assassination for example, rational choice theory suggests that the perpetrator's perceptions of opportunities and constraints shape their actions. The weapon to be used (say a long-range rifle) will have been carefully chosen. But the assassin's perception of the environment will still rationally influence the action. This may include the precise time that the killing occurs, and the exact extent to which the plan is followed. In this sense, an assassin pursues a predetermined end in what he sees as a rational way, irrespective of what an outside observer may make of events (Freilich and Newman, 2019).

Specific offences, opportunity, and intervention

Concentrating on specific offences, SCP develops preventive interventions by removing opportunities for the crime to be carried out (Clarke, 2012). This takes account of variations in offences in the context in which decisions are made. Situations in which crimes occur give concrete clues to the behaviour of the criminals. They also indicate how changes in the social and physical environment could influence criminal behaviour.

In effect, with specific crime types, the opportunities for crime are the characteristics of the situation. Analysts therefore identify the opportunities/situational characteristics that enable the perpetrator to successfully complete the crime. Finding these opportunities therefore points to where the offender's opportunities might be removed. Once the opportunities and intervention points are identified, preventive strategies are devised.

However, opportunity is not amorphous but is a structured feature. It can be examined using the script method to find preventative interventions. Looking at the exact situations in which crimes occur, analysts identify the opportunities that they provide for the offender to commit particular kinds of offence (Clarke, 1997). They then break down general settings into progressively smaller components, perhaps aided by collecting information from offenders, victims, police officers, and others.

This information can reveal answers to key questions. How was the crime committed? What helped it to be perpetrated? What barriers did the offender avoid or overcome? All this provides a map of the 'opportunity structure' of the crime. It allows analysts to decide the point(s) at which the offender's course of action can be stopped (Clarke, 2012; Freilich and Newman, 2016).

SCP strategies and techniques of crime prevention

Strategies and techniques

Five general strategies comprise the SCP framework, each embedding five crime reducing techniques (Cornish and Clarke, 2003). There are 'hard' and 'soft' interventions. Hard interventions can in a sense 'deter' offenders from committing the offense; or can make committing the crime impossible, irrespective of the offender's intent or level of motivation. Soft interventions reduce the situational prompts that increase a person's motivation to commit a crime during specific types of events (Freilich and Chermak, 2009).

The five general strategies in SCP are: increase the effort, increase the risks, reduce rewards, reduce provocations, and remove excuses. Each strategy is associated with five opportunity reducing techniques.

Techniques to **increase the effort** of perpetrators are 'target harden', 'control access to facilities', 'screen exits', 'deflect offenders' (reducing options), and 'control tools/weapons'. Examples of hardening targets are using tamper proof packaging to prevent drugs being interfered with. In homicide, a potential victim might be guarded or removed to another location. Controlling access to facilities can involve baggage screening at an airport or an office building; or having barriers with security staff in a transport network. Screening exits may suggest having documents allowing items to be exported or having security alarms at store exits to prevent stealing. Examples of reducing the options available to offenders are closing off streets and other security perimeters. Controlling tools/weapons includes the use of smart guns and legislation restricting the sale and purchase of firearms.

Turning to **increasing the risks**, techniques are 'extend guardianship', 'assist natural surveillance', 'reduce anonymity', 'utilise place managers' and 'strengthen formal surveillance'. Extending guardianship might involve setting up a neighbourhood watch scheme. An example of assisting natural surveillance is giving support to whistle blowers. These may be workers alerting authorities to concerns about a colleague, or relatives contacting police with worries about the potential violence of a family member. Reducing anonymity might include driver identification details in a taxi, or a company telephone number displayed on a delivery vehicle. Utilising place managers can imply rewarding vigilance perhaps to prevent theft in a shopping centre. Formal surveillance could involve using red light cameras.

Techniques that **reduce rewards** to the perpetrator are 'conceal targets', 'remove targets', 'identify property', 'disrupt markets', and 'deny benefits'. Concealing targets might involve using unmarked bullion trucks. An example of removing targets is using refuges for vulnerable people at risk of domestic violence. Identifying property may include marking possessions so that if stolen they can be positively identified if recovered. Disrupting markets could involve controlling classified advertisements by checking any dubious content and declining to publish it. Denying benefits to the perpetrator might include graffiti cleaning.

Turning to **reduce provocations**, techniques comprise 'reduce frustrations and stress', 'avoid disputes', 'reduce emotional arousal', 'neutralise peer pressure', and 'discourage imitation'.

Reducing frustrations and stress might include providing efficient service. An example of avoiding disputes is to construct separate enclosures in arenas for rival sports fans. Reducing emotional arousal can imply controlling or censoring violent pornography. Neutralising peer pressure could involve dispersing troublemakers in schools and other institutions. An instance of discouraging imitation is police or the media restricting publication of details of the modus operandi of a crime.

Removing excuses comprises techniques to 'set rules', 'post instructions', 'alert conscience', 'assist compliance', and 'control drugs and alcohol'. Setting rules can involve agreeing harassment codes. Posting instructions could include displaying notices on private property. An example of alerting conscience is requiring passengers' signatures for customs declarations. Assisting compliance might involve providing litter bins. Controlling drugs and alcohol is helped by holding alcohol-free events.

When analysts consider preventive techniques in specific situations, they draw on empirical literature to find interventions that have already been used successfully (Clarke and Eck, 2005). This leads to the shaping of new strategies (Ekblom, 2012a). In deciding which of the suitable looking techniques will be used, those implementing them take account of practicalities such as cost, local community endorsement, and practicability (Felson and Clarke, 1997).

Evaluating SCP strategies

In some studies, crime dropped substantially following effective intervention (Perry, Apel, Newman and Clarke, 2016). To measure the effect of specified preventive measures, the script method may be used. It analyses the sequence of behaviours and events that are the result or cause of the offender's decision making. This helps to identify opportunities and intervention points, and to determine interventions. Alternatively, analysts can assess the level of crime and/or any change in the type of crime before and after an intervention. Time series analyses have been used to investigate the impact of specific measures (Hsu and Apel, 2015), some using a 'before and after' design. Indeed, time series is a way of examining whether or nor crime was 'displaced', and if so to where or to what. Issues relating to crime displacement and SCP are much discussed (Johnson, Guerette and Bowers, 2014).

In fact, another seminal work in SCP (as well as the study on boys absconding) examined the reduction of suicide in northern England following the abolition of lethal coal gas use for domestic heating (Clarke and Lester, 2013; Clarke and Mayhew, 1988). Implications of this study included providing evidence that 'blocking opportunities, even for deeply motivated acts, does not inevitably result in displacement'. People who might have killed themselves using coal gas fumes did not, by displacement, choose another way of suicide. Applied to criminology the study pointed to a strengthened case for a situational means of crime control.

SCP and severe mental disorder

Can some psychotic behaviour be predicted?

SCP implies that an offender's actions are not random and irrational so that there is some predictability to their choices or decisions, and their actions. Consequently, the relevance of SCP to offenders with severe mental disorder may initially appear constrained. This seems especially so with disorders such as schizophrenia where psychosis is central. To the extent that SCP assumes that an individual makes reasoned choices, it seems inapplicable to situations where they are experiencing a psychotic episode. A perpetrator may follow deluded reasoning such as that he is preventing someone harassing him or is saving someone who is being persecuted. But such 'reasoning' tends not to reflect the consensus of reality experienced by others. The CIA are not really trying to kill you and the person that you attack is a shopkeeper not a CIA operative.

However, total pessimism about the potential of SCP relating to offenders with severe mental disorders may be unjustified. Recall that offenders' perceptions of their needs and their perception of the opportunities presented by the environment, both contribute to how the person behaves in the situation. Even some consistency in the way an offender with psychosis behaves according to their false beliefs may allow predictability. For example, if an individual persistently expresses the false belief that his parents and siblings are trying to harm him and that he must therefore protect himself, then, if he harms anyone, it will likely be a member of his immediate family. Such perceptions and beliefs are not based on the shared reality of others, but the behaviour, to some degree, can be anticipated.

Can predictability lead to modifications of behaviour? Earlier we saw that even with people espousing an extremist ideology, researchers used responses shaped by the specific circumstances to prevent offending (Freilich and

Chermak, 2009). A situation embedded in cultural values can be modified, using this situational view of culture and ideology.

Techniques drew on guilt and shame that intervene in individual's decision making at the right time (Wortley, 1996). If behaviour related to extreme ideology can be modified, including where the beliefs are irrational, then perhaps behaviours sometimes associated with psychosis can also be changed. Key to this is whether the irrational beliefs can be empirically identified, and whether they can be manipulated to modify decision making in a specified situation.

Behaviourally orientated interventions

As already discussed, some behaviourally orientated interventions physically prevent perpetrators from offending despite their supposed motivation, thought patterns, or emotions (Cornish and Clarke, 2008, p. 41). If a family member is targeted by an individual with delusions that they are trying to harm him or her, 'hardening the target' may be a possible technique.

If this is not practicable, where the potential perpetrator and the target live together, for example, a more flexible interpretation of 'hardening the target' may be taken. Removing the potential offender to psychiatric provision may, by putting physical and personnel barriers in place, protect the potential target. Having a potential offender wear a security tag which identifies their whereabouts and legally restricting places they can visit is a further approach. This may apply where an individual with severe mental disorder has previously committed a homicide and has been detained for some years and later released but may still pose a threat to the deceased's relatives if allowed in the area where they live.

Such an approach does not depend on assumptions about the psychology of the potential offender, their agency or lack of it at a specified time, their ability to make rational choices, or whether they act hedonistically. It just stops the potential offender getting near the target. The individual inevitably 'responds' to the preventive technique by being unable to harm the target (Newman and Freilich, 2012, p. 216).

Internal dispositions and environmental triggers

Another example arises with some 'soft' SCP approaches. These do not depend upon offender rationality or agency to reduce crime. Rather they take a behavioural view of what might otherwise be called emotional propensity. These are internal 'dispositions' towards behaviours that can be provoked by certain aspects of the environment. Such dispositions, it is proposed, may remain dormant unless certain environmental conditions arise triggering the related behaviours.

An earlier example was given of publicly displayed weapons leading some individuals to become violent, apparently by provoking an internal disposition (Wortley, 2008). An individual experiencing psychosis may be believed to have an internal disposition to violence in specific environmental circumstances. This could be towards particular people such as police officers having recognised roles in society. It might relate to specific situations such as very crowded places. In such circumstances, preventive support and supervision might be provided in a half-way house or a supported living setting rather than in full-time psychiatric hospital care. Possible environmental triggers rather than supposed internal states of the individual would be the primary focus.

Evaluation

The extent to which the script method may be used with people with severe mental disorder will depend on exact circumstances. In general, the approach can analyse the sequence of behaviours and events resulting from (or caused by) offender decision making. This can point to opportunities and intervention points for possible interventions whose effects can be measured. How useful the evaluation is will relate to the issues discussed earlier around predictability, behaviourally oriented interventions, and environmental triggers for dispositions. Any supposed 'reasons' why a person with SMD wants to kill someone may be of less relevance to prevention than their ability to do so which will depend on many potentially modifiable environmental factors.

Conclusion

Situational Crime Prevention (SCP) seeks to reduce crime by analysing the circumstances engendering specific kinds of crime. Recognising that certain situations and settings provide opportunities to commit offences, SCP uses modifications to the environment and to the management of situations to change how opportunity is structured for the crimes to occur.

Turning to aspects of SCP, its techniques imply that an offender has certain tendencies and acts in particular ways, that individuals behave rationally and make rational choices, that they can act independently, and that they behave hedonistically. SCP takes a behavioural view of people's actions, and views what otherwise might be seen as emotional states as 'internal dispositions'. SCP can take account of subculture in using preventive techniques in specified circumstances, where the values and beliefs involved are empirically identifiable, and can be manipulated to modify decision making in a specific situation.

SCP was developed by Ron Clarke, a research officer at the Kingswood Training School, Bristol, England, a boarding school for delinquent boys. In one of his seminal studies, Clarke, looking at absconding, examined the situations in which these events occurred and realised that by altering situational features absconding could be reduced.

Features of SCP include behavioural approaches and 'scripts' which help researchers analyse and understand the expectations around certain situations. The location of crime, and products and services can be designed and modified to deter crime. An assumption that offenders made rational choices in committing crimes is used to develop deterrent strategies. Concentrating on specific offences, SCP develops preventive interventions by removing opportunities for the crime to be carried out.

Five general strategies of SCP are each associated with five opportunity reducing techniques. To increase the effort of perpetrators, strategies include 'target harden' and 'control tools/ weapons'. Increasing the risks includes 'reducing anonymity' and 'strengthening formal surveillance'. Among techniques to reduce rewards to the perpetrator are 'remove targets' and 'deny benefits'. Regarding reduce provocations, techniques include 'reduce frustrations and stress', and 'discourage imitation'. Remove excuses concerns 'set rules', 'post instructions', 'alert conscience', 'assist compliance' and 'control drugs and alcohol'.

Issues important in seeking to apply SCP to homicide perpetrated by individuals with severe mental disorder include the predictability of psychotic behaviour, 'hard' behavioural interventions, and environmental triggers.

Suggested activities

Consult the website of the Arizona State University Center for Problem Oriented Policing https://popcenter.asu.edu/problems

Look at examples from their list of *Problem Specific Guides*. These include a guide on 'People with Mental Illness' (No. 40) https://popcenter.asu.edu/ sites/default/ files/ people_with_mental_illness.pdf. There are other useful guides such as on general evaluation. You get a clear view of the structure of the guides if you download the PDF.

Consider the typical patterns in approaches to problem orientated policing. These include defining and identifying the problem/crime, analysing its situational aspects, identifying approaches that reduce offending, and evaluating results.

Key text

Tilley, N. and Farrell, G. (Eds) (2012) *The Reasoning Criminologist: Essays in Honour of Ronald V. Clarke*. New York: Routledge.

This book comprises various essays highlighting the contributions of SCP to policing, product design, and other matters.

References

Agnew, R. (2001) 'Strain theory' in McLaughlin, E. and Muncie, J. (Eds) *The Sage Dictionary of Criminology*. London, Sage.

Arizona State University Center for Problem Oriented Policing (various dates) *Problem Specific Guides*. https://popcenter.asu.edu/problems.

Armitage, R. (2000) *An Evaluation of Secured by Design Housing within West Yorkshire: Briefing Note 7/00*. London, Home Office.

Becker, H. ([1963]/2008) *Outsiders: Studies in the Sociology of Deviance.* New York, Free Press.

Bowers, K. and Johnson, S. (2005) 'Using publicity for preventive purposes' in Tilley, N. (Ed.) *Handbook of Crime Prevention and Community Safety.* Portland, OR, Willan Publishing.

Braga, A. and Kennedy, D. (2012) 'Linking situational crime prevention and focused deterrence strategies' in Tilley, N. and Farrell, G. (Eds) *The Reasoning Criminologist: Essays in Honor of Ronald V. Clarke.* New York, Routledge.

Brantingham, P. J. and Brantingham, P. L. (Eds) (1981) *Environmental Criminology.* Beverly Hills, CA, Sage.

Clarke, R. V. (1967) 'Seasonal and other environmental aspects of absconding by approved school boys' *British Journal of Criminology* 7, 195–202.

Clarke, R. V. (1980) 'Situational crime prevention: Theory and practice' *British Journal of Criminology* 20, 1, 136–147.

Clarke, R. V. (Ed.) (1997) *Situational Crime Prevention: Successful Case Studies* (2nd edition). Monsey, NY, Criminal Justice Press.

Clarke, R. V. (2012) 'Opportunity makes the thief. Really? And so what? *Crime Science* 1, 3, 1–3.

Clarke, R. V. (2018) 'The theory and practice of situational crime prevention' *Criminology and Criminal Justice Oxford Research Encyclopaedias.* On-line publication January 2018. https://oxfordre.com/criminology/view/10.1093/acrefore/9780190264079.001.0001/acrefor e-9780190264079-e-327#acrefore-9780190264079-e-327-div2-3.

Clarke, R. V. and Eck, J. (2005) *Crime Analysis for Problem Solvers in 60 Small Steps.* Washington, DC: Office of Community Oriented Policing Services, United States Department of Justice.

Clarke, R. V. and Lester, D. (2013) *Suicide: Closing the Exits* (2nd edition). London, Routledge.

Clarke, R. V. and Mayhew, P. (1988) 'The British Gas suicide story and its criminological implications' *Crime and Justice* 10, 79–116. www.jstor.org/stable/1147403.

Cordner, G. (2006) *People with Mental Illness* (Guide No. 40) Arizona State University Center for Problem Oriented Policing. https://popcenter.asu.edu/content/p eople-mental-illness.

Cornish, D. (1994) 'The procedural analysis of offending and its relevance for situational prevention' *Crime Prevention Studies* 3, 151–196.

Cornish, D. and Clarke, R. (2002) 'Analyzing organized crimes' in Piquero, A. R. and Tibbetts, S. G. (Eds) *Rational Choice and Criminal Behavior: Recent Research and Future Challenges.* New York: Routledge (pp. 41–63).

Cornish, D. B. and Clarke, R. V. (2003) 'Opportunities, precipitators, and criminal decisions: A reply to Wortley's critique of situational crime prevention' *Crime Prevention Studies* 16, 41–96.

Cornish, D. B. and Clarke, R. (2008) 'The rational choice perspective' in Wortley, R. and Mazerolle, L. (Eds) *Environmental Criminology and Crime Analysis.* Portland, OR: Willan Publishing (pp. 21–47)

Cozens, P. (2008) 'Crime prevention through environmental design' in Wortley, R. and Mazerolle, L. (Eds) *Environmental Criminology and Crime Analysis.* Portland, OR: Willan Publishing (pp. 153–177).

Ekblom, P. (2012a) 'Happy returns: Ideas brought back from situational crime prevention's exploration of design against crime' Tilley, N. and Farrell, G. (Eds) *The*

Reasoning Criminologist: Essays in Honour of Ronald V. Clarke (pp. 52–64). New York, Routledge.

Ekblom, P. (Ed.) (2012b) *'Design against crime: Crime proofing everyday products' Crime Prevention Studies* Vol. 27. Boulder, CO, Lynne Rienner Publishers.

Felson, M. and Clarke, R. V. (1997) 'The ethics of situational crime prevention' in Newman, G. R., Clarke, R. V. and Shoham, S. G. (Eds) *Rational Choice and Situational Crime Prevention*. Aldershot, Ashgate.

Freilich, J. D. and Chermak, S. M. (2009) 'Preventing deadly encounters between law enforcement and American far-rightists' *Crime Prevention Studies* 25, 141–172.

Freilich, J. D. and Newman, G. R. (2016) 'Transforming piecemeal social engineering into "grand" crime prevention policy: Toward a new criminology of social control' *Journal of Criminal Law and Criminology* 105, 1, 209–238.

Freilich, J. D. and Newman, G. R. (2019) 'Situational Crime Prevention' *Oxford Research Encyclopaedias* (Criminology and Criminal Justice). http://oxfordre.com/criminology/view/10.1093/acrefore/9780190264079.001.0001/acrefore-9780190264079-e-3.

Garland, D. (2000) 'Ideas, institutions and SCP' in von Hirsch, A.et al. (Eds) *Ethical and Social Perspectives on Situational Crime Prevention*. Oxford, Hart Publishing.

Hirschi, T. (1969) *The Causes of Delinquency*. Berkley, CA, University of California Press.

Hsu, H. Y. and Apel, R. (2015) 'A situational model of displacement and diffusion following the introduction of airport metal detectors' *Terrorism and Political Violence* 27, 1, 29–52.

Johnson, S. D., Guerette, R. T., and Bowers, K. (2014) 'Crime displacement: What we know, and what we don't know, and what it means for crime reduction' *Journal of Experimental Criminology* 10, 549–571.

Kohlberg, L. (1978) 'Revisions in the theory and practice of mental development' in Damon, W. (Ed.) *New Directions in Child Development: Moral Development*. San Francisco, CA, Jossey-Bass.

Merton, R. K. (1938) 'Social structure and anomie' *American Sociological Review* 3, 672–682.

Newman, G. R. and Freilich, J. D. (2012) 'Extending the reach of situational crime prevention' in Tilley, N. and Farrell, G. (Eds) *The Reasoning Criminologist: Essays in Honor of Ronald V. Clarke*. New York: Routledge (pp. 212–225).

Perry, S., Apel, R., Newman, G. R. and Clarke, R. V. (2016) 'The situational prevention of terrorism: An evaluation of the Israeli West Bank barrier' *Journal of Quantitative Criminology* 33, 4, 727–751.

Wilson, J. Q. and Kelling, G. L. (1982) 'Broken windows' *Atlantic Monthly* 249, 29–38.

Wortley, R. K. (1996) 'Guilt, shame and situational crime prevention' *Crime Prevention Studies* 5, 115–132.

Wortley, R. K. (2008) 'Situational precipitators of crime' in Wortley, R. and Mazerolle, L. (Eds) *Environmental Criminology and Crime Analysis*. Portland, OR: Willan Publishing (pp. 48–69).

Chapter 4

Demographics and related factors

Introduction

This chapter looks at cases of homicide from 2000 to 2020 by perpetrators with SMD, mainly from the UK and the US. Perpetrator's mental health background, and the legal outcome is examined. Also discussed are the perpetrator and victim demographics of age, gender, ethnicity, and social background/occupation and their interaction. Relationships between perpetrator and victim are considered.

Perpetrator's mental health

Schizophrenia, delusions of persecution, and psychotic episodes

Homicide perpetrators Simelane, Carter, Crook, Lewis-Ranwell, Bruce, and Bonds were all reported to have schizophrenia with delusions of persecution. Simelane experienced mental health problems from his mid-teens. He was discharged from psychiatric care in December 2012 three months before killing (Welton, 2013). Carter, an inpatient in a secure hospital, moved to a community mental health setting days before he killed (Reporter, 3 April 2006). Crook was 'sectioned' in 2002 (BBC News, 20 July 2015). Lewis-Ranwell acted increasingly irrationally prior to his killings (Morris, 2019). Bruce was diagnosed with schizophrenia in 2005 after a series of violent incidents (Bernstein and Koppel, 2008). Bonds' girlfriend told investigators he was 'irrational and erratic' while off his medication, and informed emergency services on the night he killed that he was 'unhinged'. Delusions of persecution may have driven his previous assault on a police officer and anti-police social media posts (Celona and Golding, 2017).

Thaiday believed that she was 'the chosen one' and ten days before killing, was heard telling herself, 'I have the power to kill people'. Although not formally diagnosed, she may have had schizophrenia triggered by long-term cannabis use (Australian Associated Press, 2017). Dixon was diagnosed with symptoms of schizophrenia and mania (NHS England, 2013). Atkins had had schizophrenia

DOI: 10.4324/9781003172727-5

for 18 years and gave up work following a relapse (Savill, 2001). Years before killing a child in her care, Bobokulova received clinic treatment for schizophrenia (TASS, 2016). Davydov was being treated as a psychiatric patient with schizophrenia and was refusing his medication (Barr, Londoño and Morse, 2006). Harris also had schizophrenia (Reporter, 2 August 2007).

In the six months prior to him killing, Nandap experienced delusions of persecution and hallucinations, and was treated in Nigeria for psychosis (Evans, 2018). In July 2004, Wright's general practitioner found him to be 'anxious and paranoid' and referred him to a hospital mental health unit. Months later Wright told his physician that he heard voices and could alter the weather by changing his clothes (Twomey, 2009).

At his family's request, Devanov was 'sectioned' at a psychiatric unit and released seven months before killing. He believed he was Jesus Christ and was sent to create a new Jerusalem, and heard voices commanding him to kill (Gilligan, 2013). In 2018, Lacey 'disappeared' in London, deludedly believing his phone was hacked and that he would imminently die (Docking, 2018). Schloser suffered postpartum depression and had psychotic episodes for which she was hospitalised (Joyner, 2004). Soon after beginning to study law, West experienced mental disorder and was hospitalised for brief periods, eventually leaving law school. Between 1990 and 2000 psychotic episodes derailed her attempts to continue her studies (Teetor, 2002).

Other disorders

From 2002, Diaz complained of many ailments, frequently visiting doctors, or alternative therapists, and believed she had infected her children (Ellis and Emily, 2006). Schloser had a history of postpartum depression as well as psychotic episodes. When Davis killed in 2003, he was diagnosed with depression, alcohol dependence, and social anxiety, and his diary recorded plans to become a serial killer (BBC News, 15 December 2003). Laney developed odd beliefs not necessarily indicating mental disorder. A year before killing her children, she told fellow church members that the world was ending, and that God had ordered her to get her house in order (Falkenberg, 2003).

Less specific mental health problems

Prior to killing, Attias seemingly had mental health and drug problems (Lagos, 2002). Addy apparently experienced an unrecognised mental disorder for a year before he killed (Milwaukee County Case 2003CF001468). Nathan Jones' father testified in court about his son's declining mental health (Reporter, 18 December 2007). Known to police, probation, mental health, and drug support services, between February 2011 and July 2012, Tyler had four mental health assessments but was not diagnosed with a specific condition (BBC, 27 March 2013).

Identified mental disorder and general mental health issues

Reports mentioned sometimes overlapping disorders or symptoms. These were schizophrenia (Lewis-Ranwell, Bobokulova, Simelane, Carter, Harris, Crook, Davidov, Dixon, Brice, Atkins); delusions of persecution (Lewis-Ranwell, Bonds, Nandap, Simelane, Carter, Crook, Bruce, Wright); psychosis including hallucinations (Lacey, Nandap, Devanov, Laney, Thaiday, Dixon, Schlosser, West); depression (Schloser, Davis) and mania (Dixon).

In nearly all the cases, courts decided (or evidence indicated) that the perpetrator was not fully responsible for homicide because of SMD. A preponderance of schizophrenia, delusions of persecution, and psychotic episodes including hallucinations is therefore unsurprising. Other conditions occasionally identified or suspected were depression and mania. Rarely indicated were obsessive fear and psychosomatic disorders (Diaz), social anxiety (Davis), and odd beliefs not necessarily indicating SMD (Laney). Sometimes there were general mental health concerns, although no identified condition (Attias, Addy, Jones, and Tyler).

Other features of cases

History of violence

Michael Harris who stabbed his friend Carl James had previously had violent outbursts. Long before killing his mother, Bruce turned a gun on his father and two friends while hunting, and later attacked his father again. Nandap was arrested after wielding a knife on a London street, months before killing Jeroen Ensink. Simelane had several criminal convictions including for two knife offences.

Bonds had previously assaulted a police officer and posted anti-police social media rants. The day before killing his mother, Lacey attacked his father and his half-brother. Wright, two days before killing his former partner Colette Lynch, threatened to kill her brother. Hours later he forced his way into Lynch's home, attacked her, and threatened to cut her throat. Overall, violence can occur months before a killing or much closer to the event.

Abuse of drugs including alcohol

Thaiday may have developed schizophrenia triggered by long-term cannabis use. Harris smoked skunk cannabis heavily, exacerbating his schizophrenia. Nandap'a heavy use of cannabis worsened his mental disorder. Devanov seemingly took cocaine and LSD. Davis was diagnosed with alcohol dependence. Attias apparently had a history of drug problems and after killing pedestrians with his car, had blood tests indicating the presence of marijuana and Lidocaine, but these were not deemed influential in the incident.

Perpetrator declining to take medication

Crook, having been hospitalised and later discharged, refused contact with mental health services, and declined his medication. Davydov had schizophrenia and, refusing to take his medication, may have argued with his victim, psychiatrist Wayne Fenton, about it. Jones was not taking his prescribed medicines at the time that he stabbed his mother.

Initial episodes and patterns of illness

Sometimes, there is a long history of SMD as with Atkins who had experienced schizophrenia for 18 years. Other perpetrators were experiencing their first or an early episode of SMD, or the indications appeared in the few months before their killing.

Signs of Nandap's deteriorating mental health in the six months before he killed included his arrest for publicly wielding a knife, high cannabis use, strange behaviour, delusions of persecution and hallucinations, and treatment in Nigeria for psychosis.

Thaiday's long-term cannabis use seemingly triggered schizophrenia. Her mental state may have got worse months before the killings, but she had never been treated for mental illness.

Davis wrote in his diary plans to become a serial killer. Although at the time of the killing he was diagnosed with depression, alcohol dependence, and social anxiety, no obvious signs preceded his explosive violence. Laney told fellow church members a year before killing her children that the world was ending but apparently had no history of mental disorder. Addy may have had an unrecognised mental disorder before he killed.

With individuals having a long history of SMD, any recurrence may seem routine, making it hard to anticipate homicidal violence, while with comparatively sudden onset of SMD, signs may be missed because unexpected. See Table 4.1 (pp. 53–54).

Legal outcome in illustrative cases

Not guilty because of insanity, diminished responsibility, mental disease, or defect, or being not criminally responsible

Found 'not guilty' by reason of insanity, Lewis-Ranwell was given a hospital restriction order; Bruce was sent to a psychiatric recovery centre; Jones and Schloser were placed in psychiatric care; Diaz and Laney were committed to a State Hospital.

Simelane pleaded not guilty on the grounds of diminished responsibility and was sentenced to indefinite hospital detention. Found not guilty by reason of mental disease or defect, Addy was committed to a State Mental Institution.

Table 4.1 Diagnoses and indications of the mental health of perpetrators

Schiz = schizophrenia; Persec = delusions of persecution; Psych = psychosis including hallucinations; Manic = manic episode; Dep = depression; MHP = mental health problems usually unspecified; Drugs = history of drug abuse; Viol = history of violence; Off meds = declining to take medication

Name	Schiz	Persec	Psych	Manic	Dep	MHP	Drugs	Viol	Off meds
Lewis-Ranwell	✓	✓							
Lacey			✓					✓	
Bonds		✓						✓	
Bobokulova	✓		✓						
Nandap		✓	✓				✓	✓	
Thaiday		✓	✓						
Simelane	✓	✓							
Tyler						✓			
Carter	✓	✓							
Devanov			✓				✓		
Harris	✓						✓	✓	
Crook	✓	✓							✓
Davydov	✓								✓
Dixon	✓		✓	✓					
Bruce	✓	✓						✓	
Jones						✓			✓

Schiz = schizophrenia; Persec = delusions of persecution; Psych = psychosis including hallucinations; Manic = manic episode; Dep = depression; MHP = mental health problems usually unspecified; Drugs = history of drug abuse; Viol = history of violence; Off meds = declining to take medication

	Schiz	Persec	Psych	Manic	Dep	MHP	Drugs	Viol	Off meds
Schloser			/		/				
Davis		/		/	/	/	/	/	
Wright		/							/
Diaz			/			/			
Laney			/						
Addy						/			
Atkins	/								
Attias			/			/		/	
West			/						
Totals	10	8	9	1	2	6	6	6	3

Davidov, found guilty but not criminally responsible for the murder of Wayne Fenton, was moved to maximum-security psychiatric hospital. Facing a similar judgement, Devanov was detained in a secure psychiatric unit on Tenerife.

Second degree murder/manslaughter with diminished responsibility and insanity

In the US, Attias was convicted of four counts of second-degree murder. A week later the same jury found him legally insane and he was sent to Patton State Hospital, San Bernardino. A jury found West guilty of second-degree murder but disagreed about her sanity. Two years later, a jury found her insane and she was committed to a state psychiatric hospital.

In England, admitting manslaughter on the grounds of diminished responsibility, Nandap, Carter, and Davis were each sentenced to an indefinite hospital order at Broadmoor secure hospital. Harris and Wright were placed in psychiatric facilities in Bristol. Dixon was detained indefinitely at the secure Rampton Hospital. After killing his parents, Crook was considered unfit to stand trial because of his mental health problems. Eight years later he was found guilty of manslaughter on the grounds of diminished responsibility and detained at Rampton.

Pleading guilty to the manslaughter of his mother, Lacey was given an indefinite hospital order, being detained at the secure Ashworth Hospital, England. Atkins was convicted of manslaughter and detained in a high security psychiatric hospital.

Did not come to trial

A court judged that Thaiday was of unsound mind when she killed, and she did not stand trial but was held in a high security mental health centre in Brisbane. Bonds' killing of a police officer did not come to court as police shot him dead as he fled the scene. Tyler did not stand trial as, after killing of his mother, he committed suicide. Bobokulova was charged with murder, but found to have schizophrenia and was detained in a secure psychiatric hospital. Reports were unclear about the exact court judgement.

Homicides generally: perpetrator's gender and age

US Uniform Crime Reports (UCR) refer to the 'uniform' nature of the reporting documents across various jurisdictions (Dobrin, 2016, p. 6). The 2018 UCR homicide data provides information on the gender, age, and race of perpetrators (Federal Bureau of Investigation, 2018a; 2018b). Some figures from this database are given in different sections below. Figures cover a period of a year, apply to the US, and concern reported general homicides. The glossary cases cover a 20-year period, concern mainly the US and the UK, and relate only to SMD homicides. This limits comparisons. However, the US data provides a context for discussing SMD homicide, enabling one to explore similarities and differences.

FBI homicide data for 2018 (Federal Bureau of Investigation, 2018a) indicates that for *all* reported offenders 63.1% were male, 8.8% were female, and for 28.1% the gender was unknown. This is typical of perpetrators of homicides where men are greatly overrepresented as both offenders and, to a lesser degree, victims of homicide. Also, of offenders for whom age is known, offending peaks in several age bands between the ages of 17 and 34 years (Ibid.). Again, this is typical as perpetrators of homicide tend to be neither excessively young nor elderly.

SMD perpetrator's gender and age

Table 4.2 provides the age ranges of perpetrators by gender. Ages range from 18 years (university freshman Attias) to 51 years (Cook). Most are aged 21 to 30 (10 cases) and 31 to 40 years (10 cases). A few are aged 18 to 20 (2 cases) and 41 to 51 years (3 cases).

Table 4.2 Age and gender of perpetrators with SMD

Age range (years)	Number (male)	Number (female)	Totals
18–20	2	0	2
21–30	9	1	10
31–40	5	5	10
41–51	3	0	3
Totals	19	6	(25)

Of the 25 perpetrators, 19 were men and 6 were women. Men were aged from 18 to 51 years, with most in the 21 to 30 age range. The six women included were aged from 24 (Diaz) to 39 years (Laney), with five aged 31 to 40, and one in the 21 to 30 years range.

This picture for perpetrators with SMD mirrors homicides generally where younger age groups predominate. However, although there are fewer women than men perpetrators with SMD, women with SMD are over-represented compared with general homicide figures. Studies of individuals with mental disorder who committed homicide reflect this. In Austria, women accounted for 31% of these homicides (Schanda et al., 2004) and in New Zealand, 32% (Simpson et al., 2004).

Homicides generally: Perpetrator's race

Administrative race categories can be inconsistent (Phillips and Bowling, 2012, p. 372). FBI 2018 general homicide data uses race categories of 'white', 'black', 'other', and 'unknown'. Some 29% were white, 38.7% were black or

African American, 1.9% were of 'other', and 29.5% were 'unknown' (Federal Bureau of Investigation, 2018a). A separate column categorises offenders as 'Hispanic or Latino', 'Not Hispanic or Latino', and 'Unknown'. In US Census Bureau race data for 2010 the category 'white' was 74.8% and 'black or African American' was 13.6% (Humes, Jones and Ramirez, 2011, Table 4.3). The US general homicide figures therefore suggest an over-representation of black and African American homicide perpetrators compared with the population generally.

Table 4.3 Ethnicity/nationality of perpetrators with SMD by gender

Ethnicity/Nationality	Number (male)	Number (female)	Totals
White British	9	0	9
White American	5	3	8
Black British	2	0	2
African American	1	0	1
Latina American	0	1	1
Other	2	2	4
Totals	19	6	(25)

SMD perpetrator's ethnicity/nationality

Ethnicity and schizophrenia in general

In western Europe, the incidence of psychotic disorders including schizophrenia is reported to be higher among ethnic minority groups, possibly implicating 'adverse experiences' such as 'perceptions of discrimination and exclusion' (Veling, Hoek, Wiersma and Mackenbach, 2010). In the US, racial disparities in rates of psychotic disorder diagnoses are reported. African American/Black consumers show a rate of on average three to four times higher than Euro-American/White consumers. With Latino American/Hispanics the rate is approximately three times higher than Euro-American/White consumers. There may be clinical bias in diagnosing a psychotic disorder, or sociological causes such as differential access to healthcare and willingness to use mental health services (Schwartz and Blankenship, 2014). Whether higher rates of psychotic disorders among ethnic minority groups translates into higher rates of SMD homicides for this population is unclear, and the sample discussed in this chapter does not illuminate this question.

Ethnicity and SMD

The ethnicity and nationality of perpetrators with SMD was largely white British (9) and white American (8). Remaining perpetrators were black British (2),

African American (1), Latina American (1), Uzbek, (1) Australian of Torres Straits heritage (1), Nigerian living in the UK (1), and Bulgarian living in the Canary Islands (1).

All the white British, black British, and African American examples are male. Among white Americans, three (of 8) were female, as was the sole Latina American. 'Other' ethnic/ national perpetrators comprised two females and two males. The predominance of white perpetrators with SMD reflects the majority white population in the UK and the US, the source of most of the cases. See Table 4.3.

Age ranges of black British, African American, Latin American, and 'other' groups is in the spread of 21–30, and 31–40 years, consistent with this age range being predominant for all groups. Only five perpetrators fell outside this range (2 white America, and 3 white British). See Table 4.4.

Table 4.4 Ethnicity/nationality of perpetrators with SMD by age

Ethnicity/ Nationality	Ages 18–20	Ages 21–30	Ages 31–40	Ages 31–40	Totals
White British	0	3	4	3	10
White American	2	3	3	0	8
Black British	0	1	0	0	1
African American	0	0	1	0	1
Latina American	0	1	0	0	1
Other	0	2	2	0	4
Totals	2	10	10	3	(25)

SMD and perpetrator's social background/occupation

Unemployed

Most perpetrators were unemployed. There are no reports of Lewis-Ranwell working after leaving school. Lacey had no fixed address. Simelane had been in prison and was discharged from psychiatric care only three months before he killed. Tyler, known to police, probation, mental health, and drug support services appears to have been jobless.

Devanov was a 'drifter' living rough in a derelict building on Los Christianos beach, Tenerife. Bonds used several different addresses including homeless shelters. Crook had been a British Ministry of Defence worker but was made redundant soon after being convicted of harassing a female colleague. Davydov had worked for a company that trained lifeguards but was subsequently unemployed.

Bruce had been discharged from the armed forces. Wright's mental health had grown worse. Previously a garage owner, Atkins quit work owing to his mental illness. Dixon was supported by a mental health charity. Carter had been an inpatient in a secure hospital until moving to a 'half-way house' shortly before killing a fellow resident.

Employed, student, home-based parent, and unknown

Davis gained an arts degree and was later a supermarket supervisor. Bobokulova was a nanny. Originally enrolled in law school, West could not continue because of mental health problems, and later waitressed at a restaurant.

Apparently, Nandap was a student at the London University School of Oriental and African Studies. Attias was freshman at the University of California Santa Barbara. Thaiday, Schloser, and Diaz were home-based parents. Laney home schooled her children. Media reports on Harris, Jones, and Addy are unclear about their social background and employment status. See Table 4.5.

Table 4.5 Employment status of perpetrators by gender

Employment status	Number (male)	Number (female)	Totals
Unemployed	13	0	13
Home-based parent	0	4	4
Student	2	0	2
Employed	1	2	3
Unknown	3	0	3
Totals	19	6	(25)

All the unemployed perpetrators were male. Often, lack of employment seems to relate to chronic mental health problems. Where perpetrators held jobs, they were sometimes relevant to the homicide as with nanny Bobokulova who killed the child in her care. Of the two students, Nandap stabbed a stranger and Attias killed other students (and a photography shop worker) who were strangers happening to be among the pedestrians he ran over in the University of California Santa Barbara district. The four women who were home-based parents all killed their children and included Thaiday who also stabbed her niece.

SMD single and multiple victims

There were 41 victims. Of the 25 perpetrators, 18 killed one victim. The remaining seven perpetrators killed two or more victims each. Thaiday killed seven of her own children and a niece. Attias ran over four pedestrians. Lewis-Randall killed three elderly men. Each of the remaining perpetrators killed two victims: Crook his parents, Diaz her daughters, Laney her sons, and Davis a female acquaintance and her son. Three of the seven multiple victims were children killed by their mothers.

Homicides generally: victim's age and gender

FBI 2018 homicide data provides information on the gender, age, and race of homicide victims. For males, the rounded percent distribution was 77.3% and for females it was 22.5%. Regarding 0.2% of victims, gender was unknown (Federal Bureau of Investigation, 2018b). The highest numbers and proportions of victims are those aged between 17 and 44 years and especially 20 to 29 years (Ibid.).

SMD victim's age and gender

Turning to victims of perpetrators with SMD, 11 were aged 0 to 10 years (5 boys and 6 girls) and ten (3 male and 7 female) were aged 11 to 20. Therefore, most victims (21 of the 41 total) were aged 0 to 20 years. The youngest was Margaret Schloser the 11-month-old baby daughter of Dena Schloser. Of the remaining age groups, the highest totals were the 41 to 50 age group with four (1 male and 3 female) and the 81 to 90 age group also with four (3 male and 1 female). Eight victims were age 61 or over, the oldest being 90-year-old Robert Crook. A higher preponderance of younger and older victims reflects vulnerability by age. With general homicides, child victims are most likely to be killed by their parents (Brookman, 2005, p. 187). This was also the case with the child victims of mothers with SMD.

Gender balance for victims was roughly equal with 19 male and 22 being female. There was a preponderance of females in the 11 to 20 age range (3 males and 7 females). See Table 4.6.

Table 4.6 Age ranges and gender of victims

Age range (years)	Number (male)	Number (female)	Totals
0–10	5	6	11
11–20	3	7	10
21–30	2	1	3
31–40	2	0	2
41–50	1	3	4
51–60	1	2	3
61–70	1	1	2
71–80	1	1	2
81–90	3	1	4
Totals	19	22	(41)

SMD victim's age and gender compared with the perpetrator

Victims were predominantly young or old. By contrast, perpetrators were aged 18 to 51 years and 20 of the 25 perpetrators were aged 21 to 40 years. This reflects perpetrators' physical strength compared with victims, especially children. Turning to gender, 19 victims were male and 22 were female; in contrast, perpetrators were very predominantly male (19 male and 6 female) as with general homicides.

In four instances, the perpetrator killed multiple victims both male and female. Thaiday killed three sons, four daughters and her niece, Crook killed both his parents, Davis stabbed a female acquaintance and her son, and Attias ran over three males and one female. Three other perpetrators killed more than one victim of the same gender. Lewis-Ranwell stabbed three elderly men, Diaz killed her two daughters, and Laney bludgeoned her two sons.

The remaining 18 perpetrators each killed a single victim. Of these, most were male on female killings (10), followed by male on male killings (5) reflecting the preponderance of male perpetrators. There were only two female on female killings of single victims, Bobokulova who killed a child in her care, and Schloser who killed her baby daughter Margaret. See Table 4.7 (p. 62).

Homicides generally: victim's race

Race or ethnicity statistics involve inconsistent, sometimes overlapping categories (Phillips and Bowling, 2012, p. 372). Using a basic categorisation, US 2018 data indicates that of murder victims the rounded percent distribution was 52.4% black or African American, 43.1% white, and 2.8% other races. Race was unknown for 1.6% victims (Federal Bureau of Investigation, 2018b).

SMD victim's ethnicity and nationality

Ethnicity/nationality of victims

In the SMD glossary cases, there were no black British or African American victims. The largest groups were white British and white American, reflecting the preponderance of white populations in the UK and USA where most cases came from. 'Other' ethnic groups were also large with four males and six females – a white Dutch male, and a female Russian child, and seven children of the Torres Island heritage (3 boys and 5 girls). See Table 4.8 (p. 62).

Victim's ethnicity compared with the perpetrator

In most cases (18 perpetrators and 32 victims), victim and perpetrator had the same ethnicity, perhaps reflecting ties between members of each ethnic group. In only seven cases (7 perpetrators and 9 victims) did they have a different ethnic background Relatedly, of the seven perpetrators who killed victims of a different ethnic background, five involved strangers. Bonds an African American shot a Latina

Table 4.7 Gender of perpetrator and victims

Perpetrator name	Perpetrator Gender	Victim gender
Lewis-Ranwell	M	M M M
Lacey	M	F
Bonds	M	F
Bobokulova	F	F
Nandap	M	M
Thaiday	F	M M M F F F F F
Simelane	M	F
Tyler	M	F
Carter	M	M
Devanov	M	F
Harris	M	M
Crook	M	M F
Davydov	M	M
Dixon	M	F
Bruce	M	F
Jones	M	F
Schloser	F	F
Davis	M	F M
Wright	M	F
Diaz	F	F F
Laney	F	M M
Addy	M	F
Atkins	M	M
Attias	M	M M M F
West	F	M
Totals	25	41

Table 4.8 Ethnicity/nationality of victims by gender

Ethnicity/Nationality	Number (male)	Number (female)	Totals
White British	8	8	16
White American	6	7	13
Latina American	1	1	2
Other	4	6	10
Totals	19	22	(41)

American police officer; Nandap, a black Nigerian, stabbed a white Dutch victim; Simelane, a black British perpetrator, stabbed a white British schoolgirl; Bulgarian Devanov stabbed a white British woman; Wright, a black British man, stabbed his white British former partner; and West, a white American, drove her car over a Latino American. None of the across ethnic group killings appear to involve racial or cultural motives. Indeed, West was acquitted of perpetrating a racial hate crime. Perpetrators and victims of the same ethnicity are often from the same family. A perpetrator may kill their own children or parent(s). See Table 4.9.

Table 4.9 Ethnicity of perpetrator and victim

WB = white British; BB = black British; AA = African American; LA = Latino/Latina American

Perpetrator name	Perpetrator ethnicity	Victim ethnicity	correlation
Lewis-Ranwell	WB	3 WB	Same
Lacey	WB	WB	Same
Bonds	AA	LA	Different
Bobokulova	Uzbek	Russian	Different
Nandap	Nigerian	White Dutch	Different
Thaiday	Torres Straits	7 TS heritage	Same
Simelane	BB	WB	Different
Tyler	WB	WB	Same
Carter	WB	WB	Same
Devanov	Bulgarian	WB	Different
Harris	WB	WB	Same
Crook	WB	2 WB	Same
Davydov	WA	WA	Same
Dixon	WB	WB	Same
Bruce	WA	WA	Same
Jones	WA	WA	Same
Schloser	WA	WA	Same
Davis	WB	WB	Same
Wright	BB	WB	Different
Diaz	LA	2 LA	Same
Laney	WA	2 WA	Same
Addy	WA	WA	Same
Atkins	WB	WB	Same
Attias	WA	4 WA	Same
West	WA	LA	Different
Totals	25	41	

SMD victim's social background/ occupation

The largest group of victims were children including school students (15 with 5 boys and 10 girls). Retired people comprised seven of the totals (4 men and 3 women). Reports were unclear about the background/employment status of five victims (3 men including a resident of a mental health half-way house and 2 women). Three victims were adult students (1 woman and 2 men).

Two were mental health workers (a male psychiatrist and a female mental health charity employee). The killing of a female worker by a man with schizophrenia partly reflects US findings. Knable (2017) identified 33 US cases of psychotic patients killing mental health staff between the years 1981 and 2014. Unaccompanied, young, women visiting residential facilities were at greatest risk while men with schizophrenia posed most risk.

Nine other victims came from different occupations: the four men were a social worker, busboy, academic engineer, and a photography/computer shop worker. The five women were an escort, business adviser, police officer, former nurse, and a home-based parent.

Five victims were killed while working (two males – a psychiatrist and a busboy, and three females – a mental health charity worker, a police officer, and an escort). The relatively high proportion of children/school students and retired people again indicates victims vulnerable by age. They were 22 of the 41 victims.

Victim's social background/occupation compared with the perpetrator

No victim was unemployed, but 13 perpetrators were (all male) indicating their mental health problems and sometimes violent background. Of perpetrators, four women were home-based parents while only one victim was. See Table 4.10 (p. 65).

General homicide: offender–victim relationship

In male on male homicides often the participants are acquaintances (30%) or strangers (20%) after which come friends (10%) and family members (7%) (Brookman, 2005, p. 122). However, with femicide over a half of women victims are killed by their current or former boyfriend, husband, or lover (intimate femicide). Less than 10% are killed by a stranger (Ibid., p. 141). When women kill, it tends to be intimate partners or ex-partners, and family members (their children) (Ibid., pp. 162–163).

Table 4.10 Social background/occupation of perpetrator and victim

Perpetrator name	Perpetrator background	Victim background
Lewis-Ranwell	Unemployed	3 retired
Lacey	Unemployed	Business adviser
Bonds	Unemployed	Police officer
Bobokulova	Nanny	Child
Nandap	Student	Academic
Thaiday	Home based parent	8 (7 of her own children, 1 niece)
Simelane	Unemployed	Schoolgirl
Tyler	Unemployed	Retired
Carter	Half-way house resident	Half-way house resident
Devanov	Drifter / unemployed	Retired
Harris	unclear	unclear
Crook	Unemployed former government worker	2 retired
Davydov	Unemployed	Psychiatrist
Dixon	Unemployed	Mental health worker
Bruce	Unemployed/ previously in armed forces	unclear
Jones	Unclear	Former nurse
Schloser	Home based parent	Baby daughter
Davis	Supermarket supervisor	2 unclear
Wright	Unemployed	Home based parent
Diaz	Home based parent/ Former office worker	Her 2 daughters
Laney	Home based parent	Her 2 sons
Addy	Unclear	Escort
Atkins	Former garage owner	Social worker
Attias	Adult student	3 adult students, 1 photography shop worker
West	Waitress	Bus boy
Totals	25	41

SMD perpetrator–victim relationship

In most SMD instances, there was a relationship between perpetrator and victim. These comprised family members (10), professional relationships (4), friends or acquaintances (3), and a former partner (1). There were multiple victims where the relationship was family members (4 of 10 cases) and friends or acquaintances (1 of 3 cases). In only seven examples were the perpetrator and victim strangers, two involving multiple victims.

Killings by family members

In ten cases, perpetrator and victim were related usually by blood and in one instance by marriage. Sons killed their mothers (Lacey, Tyler, Bruce, Jones) or both parents (Crook). Mothers killed their children in four cases (Thaiday – who also killed a niece, Schloser, Diaz, Laney). Atkins stabbed his son-in-law.

Professional relationship

Four killings involved a professional relationship, two of them a mental health role. Davydov killed his psychiatrist. Dixon killed a visiting mental health worker. Nanny Bobokulova killed the child in her care. Addy killed an escort that he had employed. Each of these involved a single victim.

Killings by friends or acquaintances

Three cases involved a perpetrator–victim relationship of acquaintances or friends. Carter stabbed an acquaintance who was a fellow mental health resident, Davis killed two acquaintances. Harris killed a life-long friend. Davis called at the home of Dorothy Rogers, killed her, then chased her son Michael outside and stabbed him.

Other

Wright killed his former partner at her home.

Killings by strangers

Seven cases involved strangers (Lewis-Ranwell, Bonds, Nandap, Simlane, Devanov, Attias, West). Lewis-Ranwell was able to kill multiple victims because his first killing was in a house and went unnoticed for some time allowing him to enter another dwelling and attack again. Attias killed his four victims practically simultaneously with his vehicle. See Table 4.11 (p. 67).

Conclusion

This chapter examined examples of homicides from 2000 to 2020, almost all in the UK and the US. In nearly all, the perpetrator was deemed not fully responsible for the homicide because of SMD, such as schizophrenia, delusions of persecution, and psychotic episodes. Some perpetrators had a history of violence preceding the homicide sometimes over years, and

Table 4.11 Relationships between perpetrator and victim

Perpetrator name	Perpetrator Gender	Victim gender	Relationship P to V
Lewis-Ranwell	M	M M M	Strangers
Lacey	M	F	Son/mother
Bonds	M	F	Stranger
Bobokulova	F	F	Nanny/child
Nandap	M	M	Stranger
Thaiday	F	M M M F F F F F	Mother/her children and niece
Simelane	M	F	Strangers
Tyler	M	F	Son/mother
Carter	M	M	Acquaintances (Fellow residents)
Devanov	M	F	Strangers
Harris	M	M	Friends
Crook	M	M F	Son/ parents
Davydov	M	M	Patient/psychiatrist
Dixon	M	F	Client/MH worker
Bruce	M	F	Son/mother
Jones	M	F	Son/mother
Schloser	F	F	Mother/her baby
Davis	M	F M	Acquaintances
Wright	M	F	Former partners
Diaz	F	F F	Mother/her children
Laney	F	M M	Mother/her children
Addy	M	F	Client/employed escort
Atkins	M	M	father-in-law/son-in-law
Attias	M	M M M F	Strangers
West	F	M	Strangers
Totals	25	41	

abused drugs including alcohol. A few declined to take their medication. These features reflect risk factors found in wider research. For professionals, recurrences of illness with individuals having a long history of SMD may seem unexceptional, making it hard to anticipate homicidal violence, while with sudden onset of SMD signs may be missed because unexpected. In the first scenario, careful monitoring is necessary and in the second, training and vigilance is required, enabling professionals to recognise signs such as psychosis.

Homicide perpetrators with SMD like perpetrators of homicide generally tend to be male and younger (around 20 to 40 years). Regarding race and ethnicity, US general homicide data indicates an over-representation of black and African American perpetrators. However, perpetrators with SMD were very largely white British and white American, reflecting UK and the US wider population demographics. Most perpetrators with SMD of known employment status were men who were unemployed, seemingly owing to their mental health problems. Home-based parents were all women who killed their children. Seven of the 25 perpetrators killed two or more victims each and three of these instances were mothers killing their children.

Victims of homicide in general are typically young men in their twenties. Most victims of perpetrators with SMD, were aged 0 to 20 years, 11 being under ten years old. Eight victims were aged 61 or over. This preponderance of younger and older victims reflects their vulnerability by age. By contrast, most perpetrators were aged 21 to 40 years, reflecting their physical strength compared with victims, especially children. A similar number of victims was male as were female, in contrast to perpetrators who were very predominantly male (as with general homicide).

In US homicides in general 52.4% of homicide victims were black or African American, and 43.1% were white. In SMD cases, there were no black British or African American victims. The largest groups were white British and White American, mirroring wider population demographics in the UK and USA. 'Other' ethnic groups were also large and included seven children of the Torres Island heritage. In cases of SMD, victim and perpetrator usually had the same ethnicity, perhaps reflecting close ties between members of each ethnic group. In only seven cases did perpetrator and victim have a different ethnic background. Of the seven perpetrators who killed victims of a different ethnic background, five were killings of strangers, and none indicated racial or cultural motives. Perpetrators and victims of the same ethnicity were often from the same family.

Regarding victims' social background, the largest group were children including school students (15) followed by retired people (7). Relating to the SMD of perpetrators, one victim was a resident in a mental health facility, and two were mental health workers. Five victims were killed while at work. Relatively high proportions of children and school students and of retired people (22 of the 41 victims) again indicates the victims' age vulnerability. Comparing victims and perpetrators, no victim was unemployed but 13 perpetrators (all male) were, indicating their mental health problems and sometimes background of violence. Of perpetrators, four women were home-based parents while only one victim was.

Regarding offender–victim relationships, in male on male general homicides often the participants are acquaintances or strangers, after which come friends and family members. However, in male on female killings, over a half the women were victims of intimate femicide. Fewer than 10% are killed by a stranger. Women tend to kill intimate partners or ex-partners and family members (their children). With SMD cases, there was usually a relationship between perpetrator and victim: family members (10), professional relationships (4), friends or acquaintances (3), or former partner (1). In only seven examples were the perpetrator and victim strangers. There were multiple victims where the relationship was family members (4 of 10 cases) and friends or acquaintances (1 of 3 cases) and strangers (2 of 7 cases).

Suggested activities

Select a glossary case and examine it in relation to issues discussed in this chapter. Consider the perpetrator's mental health condition and whether long term or an initial episode, and other features such as history of violence, and the legal outcome. Next review perpetrator–victim demographics and relationships and identify how they aid understanding of the case. What are the most feasible preventive measures?

Key texts

Ewing, C. P. (2008) *Insanity: Murder, Madness and the Law.* Oxford, Oxford University Press.

This book presents ten controversial examples of homicides indicating the use of the insanity defence and issues arising.

References

Australian Associated Press (2017) 'Mother psychotic when she killed eight children, Queensland court rules' *Guardian* (4 May 2017) www.theguardian.com/australia-news/2017/may/04/mother-psychotic-when-she-killed-eight-children-queensland-court-rules.

Barr, C. W., Londoño, E. and Morse, D. (2006) 'Patient admits killing psychiatrist, police say' *Washington Post* (5 September 2006) www.washingtonpost.com/wp-dyn/content/article/2006/09/04/AR2006090400430.html.

BBC News (2003) 'Mother and son killed by "psychotic"' BBC News (15 December 2003) http://news.bbc.co.uk/1/hi/england/beds/bucks/herts/3322525.stm.

BBC News (2013) 'Mental health review after Cray's Hill double death incident' BBC News (27 March 2013) www.bbc.co.uk/news/uk-england-essex-21951670.

BBC News (20 July 2015) 'Manslaughter: Timothy Crook guilty of killing parents' BBC News (20 July 2015) www.bbc.co.uk/news/uk-england-wiltshire-33599525.

Bernstein, E. and Koppel, N. (2008) 'A death in the family' *Wall Street Journal* (16 August 2008) www.wsj.com/articles/SB121883750650245525.

Brookman, F. (2005) *Understanding Homicide.* London and Los Angeles, Sage.

Celona, L. and Golding, B. (2017) 'NYPD cop-killer was a schizophrenic off his meds: Girlfriend' *New York Post* (5 July 2017) https://nypost.com/2017/07/05/nypd-cop-killer-was-a-schizophrenic-off-his-meds-girlfriend/.

Dobrin, A. (2016) *Homicide Data Sources: An Interdisciplinary Overview for Researchers* (Springer briefs in criminology). New York, Springer.

Docking, N. (2018) 'Man stabbed his mum to death and tried to kill his gran's carer in psychotic episode' *Echo* (21 December 2018) www.liverpoolecho.co.uk/ news/liverp ool-news/christian-lacey-liz-lacey-murder-15584632.

Ellis, T. M. and Emily, J. (2006) 'Child-killer to leave hospital' *The Dallas Morning News* (10 November 2006) www.pressreader.com/usa/the-dallas-morning-news/ 20061110/281552286359490.

Evans, M. (2018) 'Widow of academic stabbed to death on his doorstep demands to know why psychotic knifeman was released to kill' *Telegraph* (2 July 2018) www.telegraph. co.uk/news/2018/07/02/psychotic-killer-attacked-new-father-told-police-leave-dead/.

Falkenberg, L. (2003) 'Closing arguments begin in Texas mother's murder trial' *Associated Press* (3 April 2003) www.cephas-library.com/assembly_of_god/ assembly_of_ god_member_killed _her_sons.html.

Federal Bureau of Investigation (2018a) United States 2018 Uniform Crime reports Homicide Data 'Expanded Homicide Data Table 3 Murder Offenders by Age, Sex, Race and Ethnicity 2018' Washington DC, Federal Bureau of Investigation. https://ucr. fbi.gov/crime-in-the-u.s/2018/crime-in-the-u.s.-2018/tables/expanded-homicide-data-ta ble-3.xls.

Federal Bureau of Investigation (2018b) United States 2018 Uniform Crime reports Homicide Data 'Expanded Homicide Data, Table 2, Murder Victims by Age, Sex, Race and Ethnicity, 2018' Washington DC, Federal Bureau of Investigation. https:// ucr.fbi.gov/crime-in-the-u.s/2015/crime-in-the-u.s.-2015/tables/expanded_homicide_ data_table_2_murder victims_by_age_sex_and_race_2015.xls.

Gilligan, A. (2013) 'Truth about dangerous mental patients let out to kill' *The Telegraph* (5 October 2013) www.telegraph.co.uk/news/uknews/crime/10358251/Truth-a bout-dangerous-mental-patients-let-out-to-kill.html.

Humes, K. R., Jones, N. A. and Ramirez, R. R. (2011) '*Overview of Race and Hispanic Origin United States*' Census Bureau (March 2011) (Table 3).

Joyner, J. (2004) 'Mom cut off baby's arms' *Outside the Beltway* (23 November 2004) www.outsidethebeltway.com/mom_cut_off_babys_arms/.

Knable, M. B. (2017) 'Homicides of mental health workers by patients: Review of cases and safety recommendations' *Psychiatric Annals* 47, 6, 325–334.

Lagos, M. (2002) 'Jury finds Attias guilty of murder' *Daily Nexus* (6 June 2002) http:// dailynexus.com/2002-06-06/jury-finds-attias-guilty-of-murder/.

Milwaukee County Case 2003CF001468 *State of Wisconsin vs. Keith Michael Addy* https://wcca.wicourts.gov/caseDetail.html?cacheId=19D57A47CFCA121AB4538508 BF3315A7&caseNo=2003CF001468&countyNo=40&mode=details&offset=11& recordCount=12#summary.

Morris, S. (2019) 'Killer of three elderly Devon men found not guilty of murder due to insanity' *The Guardian* (2 December 2019) www.theguardian.com/uk-news/2019/ dec/02/killer-of-three-elderly-devon-men-found-not-guilty-due-to-insanity.

NHS England (2013) *Report to NHS England of the Independent Investigation into the Healthcare and Treatment of 'Patient P'* (Commissioned by the Former North East Strategic Health Authority) http://hundredfamilies.org/wp/wp-content/uploads/ 2013/12/ RONALD_DIXON_May06.pdf.

Phillips, C. and Bowling, B. (2012) 'Ethnicities, racism, crime and criminal justice' in Maguire, M., Morgan, R. and Reiner, R. (2012) (Eds) (5th edition) *The Oxford Handbook of Criminology*. Oxford, Oxford University Press (Chapter 8).

Reporter (3 April 2006) 'Paranoid schizophrenic Marc Carter jailed for Bristol Samurai sword killing of Gino Nelmes' *HuffPost* (1 February 2013 and updated 3 April 2013) www.huffingtonpost.co.uk/2013/02/01/pranoid-schizophrenic-man2599343.html.

Reporter (2 August 2007) 'Schizophrenic addicted to skunk cannabis killed best friend' *Evening Standard* (2 August 2007) www.standard.co.uk/news/schizophrenic-addicted-to-skunk-cannabis-killed-best-friend-6602755.html.

Reporter (18 December 2007) 'Jones found not guilty by reason of insanity' *The Connection* (18 December 2007) www.connectionnewspapers.com/ news/2007/ dec/ 18/jones-not-guilty-by-reason-of-insanity/.

Savill, R. (2001) 'Son-in-law stabbed to death in marital bed' *The Telegraph* (6 June 2001) www.telegraph.co.uk/news/uknews/1311615/Son-in-law-stabbed-to-death-in-marital-bed.html.

Schanda, H., Knecht, G., Schreinzer, D., Stompe, T., Ortwein-Swoboda, G. and Waldhoer, T. (2004) 'Homicide and major mental disorders: A 25-year study' *Acta Psychiatrica Scandinavica* 110, 98–107.

Schwartz, R. C. and Blankenship, D. M. (2014) 'Racial disparities in psychotic disorder diagnosis: A review of empirical literature' *World Journal of Psychiatry* 4, 4, 133–140.

Simpson, I. A. F., McKenna, B., Moskowitz, A., Skipworth, J. and Barry-Walsh, J. (2004) 'Homicide and mental illness in New Zealand 1970–2000' *British Journal of Psychiatry* 185, 394–398.

TASS (29 February 2016) 'The murder of a child in Moscow: Investigation progress and public reaction' TASS (29 February 2016) https://tass.ru/proisshestviya/2706157 (in Russian).

Teetor, P. (2002) 'Prelude to a death' *Los Angeles Times* (5 May 2002) www.latimes.com/archives/la-xpm-2002-may-05-tm-41435-story.html.

Twomey, J (2009) 'Fury after psychotic killer walks free after four years' *Express* (22 April 2002) www.express.co.uk/news/uk/96406/Fury-as-psychotic-killer-walks-free-after-4-years.

Veling, W., Hoek, H. W., Wiersma, D. and Mackenbach, J. P. (2010) 'Ethnic identity and the risk of schizophrenia in ethnic minorities: A case-control study' *Schizophrenia Bulletin*, 36, 6, 1149–1156 (November 2010) https://academic.oup.com/schizophrenia bulletin/ article/36/6/1149/1891158.

Welton, B. (2 October 2013) 'Birmingham bus killer Philip Simelane to be held at a psychiatric unit indefinitely' *Manchester Evening News* (2 October 2013) www.manchestereveningnews.co.uk/news/uk-news/birmingham-bus-killer-phillip-simelane-6128265.

Part 2

Prevention

Chapter 5

Research into homicide and SMD

Introduction

This chapter concerns research on violence and homicide in relation to SMD (especially relating to disorders involving psychosis) and focusing on potentially preventive research. Examples of general risk factors such as poverty associated with later violence, are discussed, and the interaction of such factors with SMD. The chapter examines research into trends in the number of SMD homicides, and the possible influence of deinstitutionalisation. Also considered is the increased risk of homicide where an offender has SMD. Types and aspects of SMD are discussed in relation to violence: schizophrenia; early and late start offences; delusions of persecution, mis-identification, threat, and control; and hallucinations generating negative emotions and involving commands. The chapter examines procedural, compliance, and behavioural issues relating to the risk of violence: better and more focused treatment, treatment for non-compliance including not taking prescribed medication, substance abuse, a previous history of violence, and lack of contact with mental health services. Finally, difficulties of predicting violence and the role of risk factors in assessment are discussed.

General risk factors for violence and implications for SMD

Rabun and Boyer (2009) provide a summary of general risk factors for violence relating to demographics, personality traits, childhood factors, substance use, and behaviour history (Ibid., pp. 336–338, and list p. 341). In evaluating the risk of violence, as well as individual circumstances, general features are also considered. This is because such features, in applying to people broadly, may interact with factors associated with SMD to cumulatively increase risk. For example, substance abuse is associated with violence generally and, in combination with SMD, presents an even higher risk (McNamara and Findling, 2008).

General childhood risk factors for violence include school truancy, low educational levels, and an impoverished social background (Joyal, Putkonen, Paavova and Tiihonen, 2004). Risk factors associated with violence in the

DOI: 10.4324/9781003172727-7

general population include weak social supports, substance abuse, and poverty. These also have a bearing on violence perpetrated by individuals with SMD (Fisher, Silver and Wolff, 2006; Junginger, Claypoole, Laygo and Crisanti, 2006). Similar sociological factors effecting homicide rates in the general population also influence homicides committed by people with SMD (Large, Smith, Swinson and Shaw, 2008). A previous history of violent behaviour is a strong indicator of violence (Meehan et al., 2006).

Deinstitutionalisation and homicides perpetrated by people with SMD

Research into homicides perpetrated by individuals with SMD has examined whether their occurrence has changed over time. This is sometimes discussed in connection with deinstitutionalisation, the trend in policy in many countries to reduce the number and capacity of long-stay residential psychiatric hospitals.

Several of the studies considered in this chapter indicate the risk of homicide associated with mental disorder using odds ratios (ORs), a statistic showing association. For example, if a mental disorder, say schizophrenia, increases the risk of homicide 16 times the OR will be 16.0. After these figures, two numbers are usually given indicating the range with which one can have a 95% confidence that they are the lowest and highest values of the OR. In the German study described immediately below, the increased risk of homicide associated with schizophrenia for one group was 12.7 times. This is represented as OR 12.7 and a 95% confidence interval of 11.2–14.3.

As well as shedding light on the effects of deinstitutionalisation, the studies raise other issues that are discussed later in the chapter.

Germany

A German study noted that people with schizophrenia had an increased risk of homicide compared with the population generally. It considered whether this was associated with implementing a policy of deinstitutionalisation (Erb, Hodgins, Freese, Müller-Isberner and Jöckel, 2001). Researchers compared data on two groups of people with schizophrenia who had attempted or had committed homicide. The first group was a recent cohort in the German state of Hessen between 1992 and 1996, while the second group was a less recent cohort in the Federal Republic of Germany from 1955 to 1964.

Schizophrenia increased the risk of homicide 16.6 times (OR 16.6 and 95% confidence interval of 11.2–24.5) in the more recent cohort. In the less recent group, the increased risk was 12.7 times (OR 12.7 and 95% confidence interval of 11.2–14.3). The ORs of the two groups were not statistically different. Researchers concluded that there was no increase in the risk of homicide among people with schizophrenia since deinstitutionalization had been implemented.

Examining the more recent period, researchers found that homicide was associated with first episode acutely psychotic patients who were not using mental health services; and with chronic high-risk patients where there was a lack of 'appropriate services'. They therefore suggested that the risk of homicide could be reduced by providing specialized long-term care to those with schizophrenia at high risk for violent behaviour; and by improving the use of mental health services by acutely psychotic people (Erb, Hodgins, Freese, Müller-Isberner and Jöckel, 2001).

England and Wales

In England and Wales, researchers examined whether the rates of homicide by people with 'mental disorder' changed over time (Large, Smith, Swinson and Shaw, 2008). They compared this data with changes in the rates of other homicides in England and Wales. The study looked at four sets of official homicide statistics from 1949 to 2004. It found that the rate of total homicide and the rate of homicide perpetrated by those with mental disorder rose steadily up to the mid-1970s. After that, the rate of homicides attributed to mental disorder declined to low levels, while other homicides continued to rise.

It was suggested that the earlier rise in homicides associated with both mental disorder and other homicides related to similar sociological factors. (Presumably these continued or increased accounting for increases in homicides not connected with mental disorder). The subsequent decline in mental disorder associated homicides may have been because of improvements in 'psychiatric treatments and service organisation'. Also, there may have been an 'informal change' to the legal tests that are applied for finding that a homicide is attributed to mental disorder which may have affected the figures.

New Zealand

In a context of political concerns about deinstitutionalisation, a New Zealand study gathered information on the contribution to homicide rates of 'mental illness' (Simpson, Mckenna, Moskowitz and Skipworth, 2004). Researchers used data from government sources to conduct a retrospective study of the 1,498 homicides in the country that had occurred between 1970 and 2000. They identified, 'mentally abnormal homicide' (MAH) in which perpetrators were found unfit to stand trial, were not guilty by reason of insanity, were convicted and sentenced to psychiatric committal, or were convicted of infanticide.

The study analysed group trends and trends over time. Of the total homicides, MAH formed 8.7% with an annual rate of 1.3 per million population, which was static over the 30-year period. Total homicides increased by over 6% per year in the 20 years up to 1990, then declined in the next ten years. The percentage of MAH fell from 19.5% in 1970 to 5.0% in 2000. The researchers concluded that deinstitutionalisation 'appears not to be associated with an increased risk of homicide by people who are mentally ill'.

Overview of deinstitutionalisation

The studies considered from Germany, England and Wales, and New Zealand indicate that deinstitutionalisation appears not to be associated with an increase in the risk of homicide perpetrated by people with mental disorders. More recently published studies covering past periods when dein-stitutionalisation was implemented show a similar picture. For example, researchers reviewed a population of adult homicide perpetrators and victims in Ontario from 1987 to 2012. They examined annual rates of 'mentally abnormal' and 'non-mentally abnormal' homicide set against hospitalisation and incarceration. They concluded the declining use of psychiatric services was not associated with the rate of homicide committed by people with mental disorder (Penney, Prosser, Grimbos, Darby and Simpson, 2018).

Increased risk of homicide associated with SMD and other factors

Research has examined whether a person having SMD increases the risk that they will commit homicide. This section looks at examples of research from Austria, Sweden, and England and Wales (involving two studies – one on homicide broadly and the other concerning domestic homicide), New South Wales in Australia, and Singapore. As well as highlighting increased risk of homicide associated with SMD, the studies also raise other important issues.

Austria

A study in Austria (Schanda et al., 2004) investigated associations between homicide and 'major mental disorders' (MMD) including schizophrenia, delu-sional disorder, major depression, and bipolar disorder. Alcohol dependence and alcohol abuse were also considered. Researchers studied a 25-year period from 1975 to 1999. In total 1,087 offenders were considered who were convicted of murder or manslaughter. Of these, 961 were men and 126 were women. All defendants were seen by a psychiatrist as is customary in Austria.

The study looked at the rates of 'mitigating circumstances' arising because of MMDs among these offenders and compared these with the rates of the same disorders in the general population. MMDs were associated with an increased likelihood of homicide which was twice as much in men and six times as much in women. This increased likelihood was solely owing to schizophrenia and delusional disorder. For schizophrenia, the age-adjusted ORs in men were 5.85 (confidence interval 4.29–8.01) while in women it was 18.38 (confidence interval 11.24–31.55). For delusional disorder in men the OR was 5.98 (confidence interval 1.91–16.51).

Alcohol abuse or dependence further increased the likelihood of homicide in offenders with schizophrenia, major depression, and bipolar disorder. Researchers concluded that the increased likelihood of homicide in offenders having MMDs is not fully explained by coexisting alcoholism. They stressed the importance of ensuring 'sufficient treatment' for some types of SMD which present an increased risk of violence (Schanda et al., 2004).

Sweden

A Swedish study (Fazel, Buxrud, Ruchkin and Grann, 2010) examined the medical records of hospital patients with schizophrenia and other psychoses. These patients had been discharged and gone on to commit homicide according to the national crime register. Using a case-control design, the researchers looked at 47 instances where the patients killed within six months of being discharged, and 105 patient controls who did not commit homicide or any other violent act. Information was gathered for the period 1988 to 2001. Researchers examined factors associated with such homicides. Details of the diagnoses of the patients were obtained from the Hospital Discharge Register while the Swedish National Crime Register provided conviction information.

The study presented odds ratios (ORs) for factors associated with the 'homicide group'. These included:

- previously having been hospitalised for a violent episode (OR 5.7, 95% confidence interval 1.7–18.7),
- poor self-care (OR 5.0, 95%, confidence interval 1.5–16.7),
- not complying with medication requirements after being discharged (OR 3.8, 95% confidence interval 1.5–9.8)
- being unemployed before admission (OR of 3.3, 95% confidence interval 1.3 to 8.6),
- alcohol or other drug misuse after being discharged (OR 3.2, 95% confidence interval 1.3–7.8)
- the main reason for admission being violence or self-harm (OR 2.0, 95% confidence interval 0.9–4.1)

Researchers suggested that some factors associated with homicide relating to schizophrenia and other psychoses are potentially treatable. Substance misuse and compliance with treatment after discharge could respond to therapeutic interventions (Ibid.).

England and Wales (homicide and schizophrenia)

In England and Wales, a study described the rates of schizophrenia in a national sample of individuals convicted of homicide between 1995 and 1999 (Meehan et al., 2006). Researchers also outlined the group's social and clinical characteristics, aspects of their mental state, details of their offences, and the legal court outcome. Homicide data came from a national clinical survey. Data on individuals having schizophrenia or other delusional disorders was provided by psychiatric reports and questionnaires.

A total of 1,594 people was convicted of homicide of which 85 (5%) had schizophrenia. Of these 85 individuals with schizophrenia, 24 (28%) had had no previous contact with psychiatric services. This left 61 individuals with schizophrenia and data was available for 57 of them. Focusing on the 57 people with schizophrenia for whom data was available, 32 (56%) had been ill for less than a year. Also, 32 (56%) had shown a change in their delusional beliefs in the month before the killing. These changes were in the quality, intensity, or conviction of the delusions, or changes in the emotional response to them. The researchers suggest that regular assessment of delusions may help to detect an increased risk of violence, including homicide. Also, more provision for intensive care should be available for patients with a history of schizophrenia and previous violence.

England and Wales (mental disorder and domestic homicide)

A study examined domestic homicide and mental disorder in England and Wales (Oram, Flynn, Shaw, Appleby and Howard, 2013). It found that about 10% of convicted domestic homicide perpetrators had symptoms of mental disorder at the time. Most perpetrators including ones having mental illnesses were not in contact with mental health services in the year before the killing.

Researchers suggested that homicide risk could be reduced by initiatives encouraging individuals with mental health problems to access mental health services; and developing closer interagency working (between services for mental health and for domestic violence, police, and social services).

New South Wales, Australia

A review was made of homicides perpetrated in New South Wales, Australia between 1993 and 2002, by individuals while they were experiencing psychotic illness (Nielssen, Westmore, Large and Hayes, 2007). Case series were taken from psychiatrists' reports submitted in proceedings in the NSW Supreme Court. This showed the perpetrators' demographic and clinical features; and gave an estimated frequency of homicide occurring during psychotic illness.

In the period under consideration, at least 80 people were charged with 93 homicide offences committed during the acute phase of mental illness. High rates of drug misuse were reported, especially of substances inducing psychotic illness. Certain symptoms were 'strongly associated' with a fatal assault. These were evolving auditory hallucinations and delusional beliefs that convinced the individual they were endangered. Most victims were family members or close associates, with only nine being strangers (including three fellow patients). Most fatal attacks (69%) happened during the perpetrator's first year of illness. The first episode of psychotic illness carried the greatest risk of homicide.

Singapore

In Singapore, a study looked at 110 individuals charged with murder from 1997 to 2001, all of whom received a psychiatric assessment (Koh, Gwee and Chan, 2006). Researchers examined social/demographic data, psychiatric diagnoses, offence and victim profiles, and court outcomes obtained from prison records and psychiatric files. Offenders were mostly unmarried men aged 20 to 39 years and had a secondary school level of education or less. Depressive disorders accounted for 9.1% of the accused persons, and schizophrenia, 6.4%. Alcohol abuse and dependence disorders formed the largest diagnostic group.

Researchers concluded that perpetrators of murder have an increased incidence of psychiatric disorders. They suggested that the Singapore homicide rate may be cut through reducing factors linked to the aetiology of homicide, for example the use illicit substances and alcohol.

Types of mental disorders and features

This section looks at types of mental disorder and at aspects of mental disorder associated with increased risks of violence, focusing mainly on schizophrenia and aspects of psychosis. As well as schizophrenia more broadly, it discusses late-start and early-start offences.

Early start offenders are criminal offenders with schizophrenia who began offending at an early age (usually prior to diagnosis). Late-start offenders are those who commenced in adulthood (typically after the onset of their schizophrenia). Also discussed are delusions (involving persecution, misidentification, threat, and control); and hallucinations generating negative emotions, along with command hallucinations.

Schizophrenia

Psychiatric and psychological literature indicates that people with schizophrenia are at increased risk of perpetrating violence than are general members of the public (Sokya, Graz, Bottlender, Dirschedi and Schoech, 2007). A national survey of homicides occurring in a three-year period in England and Wales, showed that 5% of the offenders had schizophrenia (Meehan et al., 2006). This does not imply that individuals with schizophrenia as such have an increased potential for violence, rather the increased risk is associated with certain subgroups and with symptomatic periods (Joyal, Putkonen, Paavova and Tiihonen, 2004). The converse of this is that people can have schizophrenia with no attached risk of violence.

Individuals with schizophrenia may target family and friends. One study found that 50% to 60% of victims were the patient's family members while only 12% to 16% of victims were strangers. Most violence occurred in a place of residence rather than in a public setting (Joyal, Putkonen, Paavov and Tiihonen, 2004).

Late-start and early-start offenders

Researchers have distinguished between criminal offenders with schizophrenia who began offending at an early age (usually prior to diagnosis) and those who commenced in adulthood (typically after the onset of their schizophrenia). They suggest that criminality in 'early-start offenders' with schizophrenia is influenced as much by their life pattern of offending as by their psychiatric condition. For example, most early starters had committed a previous violent offence, and at the time of their violent act 70% of early starters were intoxicated compared with only 43% of late starters (Laajasalo and Hakkanen, 2005).

Also, 'late starters' are more likely to target family members than 'early-starters' (Laajasalo and Hakkanen, 2005).

Delusions of persecution, misidentification, threat. and control

Prior to 2013, the classifications of schizophrenia published by the American Psychiatric Association included a subtype of 'paranoid schizophrenia'. However, in 2013, guidance changed (in *DSM-5*). Delusions of persecution/ paranoia were classified as a symptom of schizophrenia rather than as a subtype which had been found to have limited stability as a diagnosis, low reliability, and poor validity. The term 'schizophrenia with paranoia' is still sometimes used where the individual experiences delusions of persecution.

Where delusions are not disorganised but rather are structured (which is common with delusions of persecution) there seems to be a greater likelihood that an individual will act on those delusions (Rabun and Boyer, 2009). More specifically, individuals with schizophrenia are more likely to act on delusions of persecution than they are any other type (Junginger, 1996). Delusions of persecution are associated with a greater risk of violence (Swanson et al., 2006) and the risk increases where a patient is distressed or frightened by persecutory delusions (Vandamme and Nandrino, 2005; Bjørkly, 2002). This may be because the individual can find no other explanation for the delusion than that it is real.

Examples of case studies and literature suggest that individuals experiencing delusions of persecution can plan their actions and hide their intentions.

They can also act in a way commensurate with their delusions, and target members of their family (Rabun and Boyer, 2009; Pontus, 2004).

Delusions of misidentification are also associated with violence. Capgras delusion named after French psychiatrist Joseph Capgras is the commonest example. It involves a belief that a relative or friend has been replaced by an identical looking imposter. However, the delusion can occur with several conditions including (as well as schizophrenia), Alzheimer's disease or dementia, and sometimes appears following brain injury. Capgras delusion can lead the patient to be 'paranoid' or hostile to the perceived stranger imposter (Rabun and Boyer, 2009).

So called 'threat/control-override delusions' involve false beliefs of threat or of being controlled by an outside source. They include delusions of thought insertion and of thought control. A belief of loss of control is considered to contribute to an increased risk of violence (Bjørkly, 2002). This view is contested but it is however accepted that such delusions can sometimes lead to violence (Appelbaum, Robbins and Monahan, 2000).

Hallucinations generating negative emotions, and command hallucinations

Some hallucinations generate negative feelings such as anger, sorrow, or irritability and are more likely to produce violent behaviour (Cheung, Schweitzer, Crowley and Tuckwell, 1997). The risk is likely to increase if the hallucination is related to a delusion (Bjørkly, 2002).

Other hallucinations concern commands. For example, the individual may hear a voice telling them to do something, perhaps to harm themselves or someone else. These commands can be compelling, and the voices seem to be convincingly 'outside' the individual who is hearing them. Where the command is to harm others, the risk of complying with it is increased in certain circumstances. These are that the patient's delusions are consistent with the theme of the hallucinations, that the voice is familiar, and that it generates negative emotions (Braham, Trower and Birchwood, 2004; Rabun and Boyer, 2009).

Treatment, procedural and behavioural issues, and homicide by individuals with SMD

In this section the focus is on better and more focused treatment, and on procedural and behavioural issues bearing on risks of violence, namely a previous history of violence, declining to take medication, substance abuse, and not having contact with mental health services.

Better and more focused treatment

The importance of suitable and timely treatment is supported by Nielssen and Large (2010) who reviewed rates of homicide and made a meta-analysis.

Homicide rate during first episode psychosis was 1.59 per 1000 (95% CI) and 0.11 per 1000 (95% CI) after treatment.

Research discussed earlier indicated the need for better and more focused treatment. A study in Germany pointed to the need for strategies to improve the take up of mental health services by acutely psychotic people; and providing specialized long-term care to individuals with schizophrenia at high risk for violent behaviour (Erb, Hodgins, Freese, Müller-Isberner and Jöckel, 2001). Austrian research (Schanda, et al., 2004) intimated that there was insufficient treatment for some types of MMD (schizophrenia and delusional disorder, major depression and bipolar disorder) presenting an increased risk of violence.

In England and Wales (Meehan et al., 2006) research indicated that individual's delusions should be regularly assessed to help detect an increased risk of violence including homicide. For patients with a history of schizophrenia and previous violence, more intensive care should be made available. Other researchers examined domestic homicide and mental disorder (Oram, Flynn, Shaw, Appleby and Howard, 2013). They proposed that homicide risk might be reduced by implementing strategies that encourage individuals with SMD to contact and use mental health services; and by developing approaches ensuring closer interagency working.

Australian research suggests that risks of violence and homicide might be reduced by regular monitoring of evolving auditory hallucinations and delusional beliefs convincing the individual that they were endangered (Nielssen, Westmore, Large and Hayes, 2007).

Previous history of violence

Earlier, the chapter examined the risk of violence. This included considering general features associated with violence because such features apply to people broadly and may interact with factors associated with SMD cumulatively increasing risk. A strong indicator of violence was a previous history of violent behaviour (Meehan et al., 2006).

A study in Sweden (Fazel, Buxrud, Ruchkin and Grann, 2010) compared patients with schizophrenia and other psychoses who killed within six months of being discharged, and 105 patient controls who did not. Factors associated with the 'homicide group' included previously having been hospitalised for a violent episode, and the main reason for admission being violence to others (or self-harm).

A history of violence can refer to incidents that occurred long before the present but can also include very recent behaviour. In cases where the violence is very recent it is important that, where services have been involved (including police, community health personnel, and hospital staff), this is communicated to other interested parties. Information about recent violence can also come from relatives and friends of the perpetrator.

William Bruce and previous history of violence

William Bruce had previously joined the armed forces but had been discharged and was apparently unemployed. He was diagnosed with 'paranoid schizophrenia' (what would now likely be identified as schizophrenia with delusions of persecution) in 2005 after a series of violent incidents. Bruce's previous violence included a 2005 near-fatal hunting accident when he turned a gun on his father and two friends following which he was admitted to Acadia Hospital, Bangor, Maine. He was sent there again in 2006 after another attack on his father and on 6 February 2006 was moved to Riverview Psychiatric Recovery Center, Augusta, Maine. He was discharged on 20 April 2006. Two months later, on 20 June 2006, believing his mother Amy to be an Al Qaeda agent, he fatally hit her with a hatchet as she sat working at her desk and deposited her body in the bathtub. Bruce's body was discovered by her husband Joe Bruce when he returned home from work on the afternoon of 20 June 2006. William Bruce was later arrested at his grandfather's house in South Portland. Bruce's father believed that his son should not have been released from Riverview Psychiatric Recovery Center in April 2006 (Bernstein and Koppel, 2008; Boston News, 2006; Novacic, 2015).

Not taking prescribed medication

Among priorities to prevent homicide by men with psychiatric disorders, providing adequate treatment and facilitating compliance with long-term treatment have been suggested (Sher and Rice, 2015). The latter includes taking prescribed medication.

A person with SMD declining prescribed medication has been associated with violence in some instances. In reports of homicides by people with SMD it is sometimes noted that the perpetrator should have been taking prescribed medication but was not doing so. Among reasons for an individual not complying are a dislike of the side effects of medication, problems with substance abuse, a poor relationship with the treating psychiatrist, and not recognising that they have a mental disorder (anosognosia).

Despite lack of insight in their mental disorder, a patient may continue to take their medication for many reasons. They may wish to please their family or their psychiatrist or may remain aware of difficulties when they have stopped taking medication before (Torrey, 2012, p. 118).

A study of individuals with schizophrenia indicated that those who did not adhere to medication prescribed were more likely to be arrested, or re-hospitalised, or to commit violent acts (Ascher-Svanum, Faries, Zhu, Furiak and Montgomery, 2006).

Earlier, the chapter considered research in Sweden (Fazel, Buxrud, Ruchkin and Grann, 2010) into whether a person has SMD increases the risk that they will commit homicide. Factors associated with the 'homicide group' included not complying with medication requirements after being discharged.

Vitali Davydov and declining to take medication

Vitali Davydov graduated from high school in 2005. He worked for a company that trained lifeguards but later was seemingly unemployed. At the age of 19, he was being treated as a psychiatric patient with schizophrenia and was declining to take his medication. On Saturday, 2 September 2006, Dr Wayne Fenton saw Davydov in consultation, with the patient's father present. Wayne Fenton was a psychiatrist with a private practice in Bethesda, Maryland.

He made an appointment to see Davydov again later in the week. On Sunday, 3 September the patient's father called Dr Fenton, asking him to immediately see his son who was angry about taking medication. At 4 pm, Dr Fenton saw Davidov in his office alone and apparently encouraged him to take his antipsychotic medicines. The father had left to run an errand. When the father returned, his son was standing outside with blood on his hands. Mr Davydov called emergency services, but Dr Fenton was declared dead at the scene. It emerged that the patient had beaten him to death using his fists (Barr, Londoño, and Morse, 2006; Simon, 3 March 2011; Wiggin, 2011)

Substance abuse

Substance abuse featured largely when the chapter considered general risk factors associated with violence and implications for people with SMD. It was among the risk factors associated with violence in the population in general and which also contribute to violence perpetrated by individuals with SMD (Fisher, Silver and Wolff, 2006; Junginger, Claypoole, Laygo and Crisanti, 2006). As well as being associated with violence broadly, substance abuse in combination with SMD is an even higher risk (McNamara and Findling, 2008).

When the increased risk of homicide associated with SMD and other factors was considered earlier, again substance abuse was a feature. An Austrian study looked at offenders with schizophrenia, major depression, and bipolar disorder. Where they also experienced alcohol abuse or dependence this further increased the likelihood of homicide. Researchers concluded that the increased likelihood of homicide in offenders having MMDs is not fully explained by coexisting alcoholism (Schanda et al., 2004).

In Sweden, a study (Fazel, Buxrud, Ruchkin and Grann, 2010) compared patients with schizophrenia and other psychoses who killed within six months of being discharged, and 105 patient controls who did not. Factors associated with the 'homicide group' included alcohol or other drug misuse after being discharged.

The review in New South Wales, Australia (1993 to 2002) identified at least 80 people charged with 93 homicide offences committed during the acute phase of mental illness. Researchers reported high rates of drug misuse, especially ones inducing psychotic illness (Nielssen, Westmore, Large and Hayes, 2007).

The Singapore research looked at 110 individuals charged with murder from 1997 to 2001, all of whom received a psychiatric assessment. While depressive disorders accounted for 9.1% of the accused persons and schizophrenia, 6.4%, it was alcohol abuse and dependence disorders which formed the largest diagnostic group (Koh, Gwee and Chan, 2006).

Criminality in 'early-start offenders' with schizophrenia appears to be influenced by both their life pattern of offending and their psychiatric condition. At the time of their violent act, 70% of early starters were intoxicated compared with 43% of late starters (Laajasalo and Hakkanen, 2005).

Torrey (2012) notes that among drugs that may particularly promote violence among some people are alcohol, amphetamines, cocaine, and phencyclidine (PCP) (Ibid., p. 180).

Not having contact with mental health services

Could risk of homicide be lessened by initiatives encouraging individuals with SMD to better use mental health services? Sometimes, when violence or homicide has been perpetrated by a person with SMD it is noted that they have not been in contact with mental health services. The implication is that if they had been then prevention might have been possible. This applies to individuals already known to have SMD. It also concerns people experiencing such disorders for the first time but who if identified might have received the required support.

When examining research on the possible effects of deinstitutionalisation, a German study was discussed. It found that homicide was associated with first episode acutely psychotic patients who were not using mental health services. The researchers suggested reducing homicides by improving the use of mental health services by acutely psychotic people (Erb, Hodgins, Freese, Müller-Isberner and Jöckel, 2001).

Among research looking at factors increasing the risk of violence with people with SMD was a study of domestic homicide and mental disorder in England and Wales (Oram, Flynn, Shaw, Appleby and Howard, 2013). It found that most perpetrators (including ones having mental illnesses) in the study were not in contact with mental health services in the year before the killing. This led to the suggestion that homicide risk could be reduced by initiatives encouraging individuals with SMD to access mental health services.

Difficulties predicting violence and the role of risk factors in assessment

Even sophisticated risk assessment tools may not help to predict violence in psychosis (Singh, Serper, Reinharth and Fazel, 2011) and may be less likely to predict homicide.

Predicting violence from a specific individual with a mental disorder can be challenging, partly because such violence is infrequent, and its overall prevalence is low (Rabun and Boyer, 2009). This is an instance of the broad observation that infrequent events are harder to predict than frequent ones. In examining possible causal links to violence, researchers have considered certain diagnoses (like schizophrenia), symptom categories (such as hallucinations), narrower symptoms (for example delusions of threat or of being controlled by an outside source), and 'static' and 'dynamic' (changeable) factors in risk assessments (Bjørkly, 2002).

It is argued that there is a role for actuarial instruments in interviewing patients with schizophrenia and assessing risk. Such instruments draw on information from research that suggests factors associated with increased risk of perpetrating violence. This helps ensure that key risk factors are considered. The approach is then refined by uncovering factors that are unique to the individual.

The overall risk assessment therefore involves actuarial data and information gathered in the interview. The clinician evaluates the general factors associated with increased risk of violence. He or she then draws out facts that are unique to the patient using these to help make a judgement. The opinion is presented as a risk assessment, not as a prediction of violence in a specific individual (Rabun and Boyer, 2009).

Where decisions about an individual's risk of violence and related matters leads to their detention and treatment, decision makers take account of potentially competing issues. These include an individual's freedom to participate in society considered alongside the safety of the general population. Where a person's estimated risk of harming someone in their care contributes to their being debarred from working with vulnerable people, account is taken of limiting an individual's freedom as well as the safety of potential clients. Evidence that is used to come to such difficult decisions needs to be thoroughly assessed.

Conclusion

General risk factors associated with later violence are considered when assessing the risk of violence of individuals with SMD. Research into homicides perpetrated by individuals with SMD over time exonerates deinstitutionalisation as a blanket policy from precipitating more homicides.

Risk of homicide increases where an offender has SMD as well as a history of previous violence, non-compliance with medication requirements, and drug and alcohol misuse. Symptoms that have been strongly associated with a fatal assault are evolving auditory hallucinations and delusional beliefs leading to the individual becoming convinced they were endangered. First episode psychotic illness has the greatest risk of homicide. Among preventive steps may be more provision for intensive care for patients with a history of schizophrenia and previous violence; ensuring that individuals with mental health problems access mental health services; and developing closer interagency working.

Concerning schizophrenia, an increased potential for violence is associated with delusions of persecution, misidentification, threat, and control; and hallucinations generating negative emotions, and command hallucinations

Regarding treatment, strategies are needed to improve the take up of mental health services by acutely psychotic people. Enough treatment is required for types of SMD with increased risk of violence. Also needed is provision of specialized long-term care to individuals with schizophrenia at high risk for violence. Strategies could better encourage individuals with SMD to use mental health services, and to ensure closer interagency working. There could be more regular monitoring of evolving auditory hallucinations and delusional beliefs that convince the individual that they are endangered.

A person with SMD declining prescribed medication can be associated with violence including homicide. Individuals with schizophrenia not complying with medication requirements may be more likely to be arrested, re-hospitalised, or to commit violent acts.

Substance abuse is associated with violence broadly and presents an even higher risk in combination with SMD. For example, offenders with schizophrenia who also experience alcohol abuse/dependence can have increased likelihood of homicide.

In examining the risk of violence, general features associated with violence are considered because they apply to people broadly and may interact with factors associated with SMD cumulatively increasing risk. A strong indicator of violence is a previous history of it. This includes having previously been hospitalised for a violent episode, and the main reason for admission being violence to others (or self-harm). In cases of very recent violence, any services involved should communicate details (including from relatives and friends of the perpetrator) to other interested parties.

Sometimes, when violence or homicide has been perpetrated by a person with SMD, they have not been in contact with mental health services, reducing the likelihood of prevention. This applies to individuals already known to have SMD, as well as first-timers who if identified might have received support. Homicide might be reduced by improving the use of these services, and by initiatives encouraging individuals with SMD to access mental health services.

Predicting violence from a specific individual with SMD is challenging, because violence is infrequent, and its overall prevalence low. Actuarial instruments used in interviewing patients with schizophrenia and assessing risk draw on research suggesting factors associated with increased risk of perpetrating violence. The patient is then interviewed to uncover unique personal factors. Both are used to help to make a risk assessment.

Suggested activities

Select a case from the glossary of the book. Use the internet and other reference to flesh out the events surrounding it. Consider your observations in the light of the research discussed in the present chapter. Were any of the issues discussed here especially pertinent? What preventive approaches might have reduced the risk of homicide?

Select a second case and carry out a similar analysis. Consider any pertinent issues and approaches that might reduce the risk of homicide. Reflect on the differences and similarities in the two cases and reflect on the reasons.

Key texts

Kasper, S. and Papadimitriou, G. N. (Eds) (2009) (2nd edition) *Schizophrenia: Biopsychosocial Approaches and Current Challenges* (Medical Psychiatry Series). New York and London, Informa Healthcare.

This edited international text has contributions from the US, UK, Europe, Africa, Australia, South Africa, and Korea. Its main parts deal with 'Diagnosis and Psychopathology', 'Neurobiology', 'Pharmacological Treatment Strategies', and 'Schizophrenia and Society'.

Rabun, J. and Boyer, S. (2009) 'Violence in schizophrenia: Risk factors and assessment' in Kasper, S. and Papadimitriou, G. N. (Eds) (2009) *Schizophrenia: Biopsychosocial Approaches and Current Challenges*. London, Informa Healthcare.

This book chapter gives an overview of some of the issues relating to violence and schizophrenia.

References

Appelbaum, P., Robbins, P. and Monahan, J. (2000) 'Violence and delusions: Data from the McArthur Violence Risk Assessment Study' *American Journal of Psychiatry* 157, 4, 566–572.

Ascher-Svanum, H., Faries, D. E., Zhu, B., Furiak, N. M. and Montgomery, W. (2006) 'Medication adherence and long-term functional outcomes in the treatment of schizophrenia in usual care' *Journal of Clinical Psychiatry* 67, 453–460. https://link.springer.com/article/10.1186/1756-0500-2-6.

Barr, C. W., Londoño, E. and Morse, D. (2006) 'Patient admits killing psychiatrist, police say' *Washington Post* (5 September 2006) www.washingtonpost.com/wp-dyn/content/ article/2006/09/04/AR2006090400430.html.

Bernstein, E. and Koppel. N. (2008) 'A death in the family' *Wall Street Journal* (16 August 2008) www.wsj.com/articles/SB121883750650245525.

Bjørkly, S. (2002) 'Psychotic symptoms and violence towards others – a literature review of some preliminary findings: Part 2: Hallucinations' *Aggression and Violent Behaviour* 7, 6, 605–615.

Boston News (2006) 'Mentally ill son charged with murdering his mother' *Boston News* (22 June 2006) http://archive.boston.com/news/local/maine/articles/2006/06/22/mentally_ill_son_charged_with_murdering_his_mother/.

Braham, L., Trower, P. and Birchwood, M. (2004) 'Acting on command hallucinations and dangerous behaviour: A critique of the major findings in the last decade' *Clinical Psychology Review* 24, 513–528.

Cheung, P., Schweitzer, I., Crowley, K. and Tuckwell, V. (1997) 'Violence in schizophrenia: Role of hallucinations and delusions' *Schizophrenia Research* 26, 2–3, 181–190.

Erb, M., Hodgins, S., Freese, R., Müller-Isberner, R. and Jöckel, D. (2001) 'Homicide and schizophrenia: Maybe treatment does have a preventive effect' *Criminal Behaviour and Mental Health* 11, 1, 6–26. www.ncbi.nlm.nih.gov/pubmed/12048536.

Fazel, S., Buxrud, P., Ruchkin, V. and Grann, M. (2010) 'Homicide in discharged prisoners with schizophrenia and other psychoses: A national case-control study' *Schizophrenia Research* 123, 263–269.

Fisher, W. H., Silver E. and Wolff, N. (2006) 'Beyond criminalization: Toward a criminologically informed framework for mental health policy and services research' *Administration and Policy in Mental Health* 33, 5, 544–557.

Joyal, C., Putkonen, A., Paavova, P. and Tiihonen, J. (2004) 'Characteristics and circumstances of homicidal acts committed by offenders with schizophrenia' *Psychological Medicine* 34, 433–442. www.researchgate.net/publication/8449447_Characteristics_and_circumstances_of_homicidal_acts_committed by offenders with schizophrenia.

Junginger, J. (1996) 'Psychosis and violence: The case for a content analysis of psychotic experience' *Schizophrenia Bulletin* 22, 1, 91–93.

Junginger J., Claypoole, K., and Laygo, R. and Crisanti, A. (2006) 'Effects of serious mental illness and substance abuse on criminal offenses' *Psychiatric Services* 57, 6, 879–882.

Koh, K. G. W. W., Gwee, K. P. and Chan, Y. H. (2006) 'Psychiatric aspects of homicide in Singapore: a five-year review (1997–2001)' *Singapore Medical Journal* 47, 4, 297–304www.smj.org.sg/sites/default/files/4704/4704a8.pdf.

Laajasalo, T. and Hakkanen, H. (2005) 'Offence and offender characteristics among two groups of Finnish homicide offenders with schizophrenia: Comparison of early- and late-start offenders' *Journal of Forensic Psychiatry and Psychology* 16, 1, 41–59.

Large, M., Smith, G., Swinson, N. and Shaw, J. (2008) 'Homicide due to mental disorder in England and Wales over 50 years' *The British Journal of Psychiatry* 93, 2, 130–133 (Published online by Cambridge University Press 2 January 2008) www.cambridge.org/core/journals/the-british-journal-of-psychiatry/article/homicide-due-to-mental-disorder-in-england-and-wales-over-50-years/ C07EACF0A07 FFAAE2995B 2B4EB7C8558.

McNamara, N. and Findling, R. (2008) 'Guns, adolescents and mental illness' *American Journal of Psychiatry* 165, 2, 190–194.

Meehan, J., Flynn, S., Hunt, I. M., Robinson, J., Bickley, H., Parsons, R., Amos, T., Kapur, N., Appleby, L. and Shaw, J. (2006) 'Perpetrators of homicide with schizophrenia: A national clinical survey in England and Wales' *Psychiatric Services* 57, 11, 1648–1651.

Nielssen, O. and Large, M. (2010) 'Rates of homicide during the first episode of psychosis and after treatment; a systematic review and meta-analysis' *Schizophrenia Bulletin* 36, 702–712.

Nielssen, O. B., Westmore, B. D., Large, M. M. B. and Hayes, R. A. (2007) 'Homicide during psychotic illness in New South Wales between 1993 and 2002' *Medical Journal of Australia* 186, 301–304. www.mja.com.au/journal/2007/186/6/homicide-during-psychotic-illness-new-south-wales-between-1993-and-2002.

Novacic, I. (2015) 'Violent minds: Standing at the crossroads of mental health, public safety' *CBS News* (16 June 2015) www.cbsnews.com/news/violent-minds-standing-a t-the-crossroads-of-mental-health-public-safety/.

Oram, S., Flynn, S. M., Shaw, J., Appleby, L. and Howard, L. M. (2013) 'Mental illness and domestic homicide: A population-based descriptive study' *Psychiatric Services* (October 2013), 64, 10, pp. 1006–1011.

Penney, S. R., Prosser, A., Grimbos, T., Darby, P. and Simpson, A. I. (2018) 'Time trends in homicide and mental illness in Ontario from 1987 to 2012: EXAMINING the effects of mental health service provision' *The Canadian Journal of Psychiatry*, 63, 6, 387–394. https://journals.sagepub.com/doi/10.1177/0706743717737034.

Pontus, A. (2004) 'Violence in schizophrenia versus limbic psychotic trigger reaction: Prefrontal aspects of volitional action' *Aggression and Violent Behaviour* 9, 5, 503–521. www.researchgate.net/publication/223057538_Violence_in_schizophrenia_ versus_limbic_ psychotic_trigger_reaction_Prefrontal_aspects_of_volitional_action.

Rabun, J. and Boyer, S. (2009) 'Violence in schizophrenia: Risk factors and assessment' in Kasper, S. and Papadimitriou, G. N. (Eds) *Schizophrenia: Biopsychosocial Approaches and Current Challenges.* London, Informa Healthcare.

Schanda, H., Knecht, G., Schreinzer, D., Stompe, Th., Ortwein-Swoboda, G. and Waldhoer, Th. (2004) 'Homicide and major mental disorders: A 25-year study' *Acta Psychiatrica Scandinavica* (5 July 2004) https://onlinelibrary.wiley.com/doi/abs/10. 1111/j.1600-0047.2004.00305.x.

Sher, L. and Rice, T. (2015) 'World Federation of Societies of Biological Psychiatry (WFSBP) Task Force on Men's Mental Health. Prevention of homicidal behaviour in men with psychiatric disorders' *World Journal of Biological Psychiatry* 16, 212–229.

Simon, R. I. (2011) 'Patient violence against healthcare professionals' *Psychiatric Times*, 28, 2 (3 March 2011) www.psychiatrictimes.com/psychiatric-emergencies/pa tient-violence-against-health-care-professionals.

Simpson, A. I. F., Mckenna, B., Moskowitz, A. and Skipworth, J. (2004) 'Homicide and mental illness in New Zealand, 1970–2000' *The British Journal of Psychiatry* 185, 5, 394–398 (Published by Cambridge University Press: 2 January 2018).

Singh J. P., Serper M., Reinharth J. and Fazel S. (2011) 'Structured assessment of violence risk in schizophrenia and other psychiatric disorders: A systematic review of the validity, reliability, and item content of 10 available instruments' *Schizophrenia Bulletin* 37, 899–912.

Sokya, M., Graz, C., Bottlender, P., Dirschedi, P. and Schoech, H. (2007) 'Clinical correlates of later violence and criminal offences in schizophrenia' *Schizophrenia Research* 94, 89–98. www.ncbi.nlm.nih.gov/pubmed/17509834.

Swanson, J., Swartz, M., Van Dorn, R., Elbogen, E., Wagner, H., Rosenheck, R., Stroup, T., McEvoy, J. and Lieberman, J. (2006) 'A national study of violent behaviour in persons with schizophrenia' *Archives of General Psychiatry* 63, 490–499. www.ncbi.nlm.nih.gov/pubmed/16651506.

Torrey, E. F. (2012) *The Insanity Offense: How America's Failure to Treat the Seriously Mentally Ill Endangers its Citizens.* New York, Norton.

Vandamme, M. and Nandrino, J. (2005) 'Temperament and character inventory in homicidal, nonaddicted paranoid schizophrenic patients: A preliminary study' *Psychological Reports* 95, 393–406.

Wiggin, K. (2011) 'Patient who killed psychiatrist now accused of slaying hospital roommate' *CBS News* (24 October 2011) www.cbsnews.com/news/patient-who-killed-psychiatrist-now-accused-of-slaying-hospital-roommate/.

Chapter 6

Situational Crime Prevention, homicide, and SMD: cases

Introduction

Four examples of homicides (2015–2020) involving perpetrators with SMD are presented: Lewis-Ranwell, Christian Lacey, Gyulchekhra Bobokulova, and Timchang Nandap. After briefly outlining Situational Crime Prevention (SCP), the chapter uses it to analyse the four cases, indicating where prevention may have been possible. Examination also shows where techniques are rendered ineffectual because of the nature of the cases, and here alternatives are discussed, sometimes involving pre-emptive action. These are: recognising and acting on indications of increased risk of violence; correctly assessing and evaluating SMD; the role of psychiatric care as protection and prevention; enhancing communications among professionals; improving training and understanding of procedures; the use of agencies and better supervision of workers with children; and controlling the abuse of drugs and internet content. Police guidance based on situational approaches reinforces and supplements some of the points raised. In all this, it is important to recognise that individuals may be reluctant to interact with people and agencies that discern risk in their behaviour.

Alexander Lewis-Ranwell

Alexander Lewis-Ranwell, 38, of Croyde, North Devon, UK was diagnosed with schizophrenia with delusions of persecution (Morris, 2019). On 9 February 2019, he was arrested and held at Barnstaple police station for a disturbance at a local farm. His mother Jill telephoned police after his arrest expressing 'grave concerns' should he be freed because he had nowhere to stay. Lewis-Ranwell was charged with burglary and released at 2.49 am when he was taken to a centre for homeless people in Barnstaple. He left the centre after threatening to kill a staff member.

A few hours later, Lewis-Ranwell threatened 82-year-old farmer John Ellis with a saw and was brought back to Barnstaple police station at 10 am. A police inspector reviewing his detention wrote that afternoon that the detainee 'potentially presents a serious risk to the public if released'. Police consulted

DOI: 10.4324/9781003172727-8

the Crown Prosecution Service about the farmer Ellis incident, jointly deciding there was insufficient evidence to bring a charge (Morris, 2019). A forensic medical examiner Dr Mihal Pichui saw Lewis-Ranwell in his cell at 6.30 pm, finding him 'not acutely unwell' and a full mental health assessment was not made (Sky News, 2019).

Next morning, 10 February Lewis-Ranwell was released and travelled to Exeter arriving in the St David's area about 12.30 pm. Stopping at a terraced house, he read a note on its door advertising that the 80-year-old resident sought a new home (Dilley and Kemp, 2019). It is reported that he deludedly believed that the occupant was holding a kidnapped girl in the cellar of the house. Lewis-Ranwell entered the terraced home and battered to death 80-year-old Anthony Paine with a hammer. A few hours later, in the city's St Thomas area, he found a garden spade, and entered a house. There he bludgeoned twins Dick and Roger Carter, aged 84, wrongly believing they were implicated in child abuse and torture (Sky News, 2019).

Following the attacks, Lewis-Ranwell slept outdoors. At 5 am he went to the Rougemont Hotel, Exeter, entered the lobby and demanded breakfast. Told he must wait, he threatened night manager Stasys Belevicius, throwing a glass bowl then wielding a knife. Police were called and the attacker was arrested and remanded in custody (Dilley and Kemp, 2019). Concerns being raised about his mental health, Lewis-Ranwell was transferred to a psychiatric unit for assessment and later detained in Broadmoor secure hospital, Berkshire (Sky News, 2019).

When the case came before Mrs Justice May, at Exeter Crown Court, psychiatrists testified that at the time of the killings Lewis-Ranwell believed his actions justified because he was rescuing people. Prosecution argued the defendant bore some responsibility. Before returning their verdict, the jury raised concerns about the 'state of psychiatric services' in Devon and 'failings in care'. Found not guilty by reason of insanity, the defendant was detained by a hospital order under the Mental Health Act (Sky News, 2019).

After the trial, Devon and Cornwall police said that (following the farmer Ellis incident) Lewis-Ranwell was released on bail so that additional enquiries could be completed to refer the case back to the Crown Prosecution Service. During his custody on 8 and 9 February 2019, Lewis-Ranwell saw several medical professionals at the police's request, but there was no recommendation for a full mental health assessment. On 9 February, a duty custody officer noted concerns about Lewis-Ranwell, and a National Health Service Liaison and Diversion Officer was telephoned who recommended that the detainee be assessed by the emergency duty team.

That team requested that Lewis-Ranwell be seen by a mental health professional. However, a Liaison and Diversion nurse was unavailable so recommended that a forensic medical examiner attend. This was arranged and police stated that the examiner observed no evidence of acute mental illness warranting admission to hospital. A custody pre-release plan was written and Lewis-Ranwell was given paperwork enabling him to access Liaison and

Diversion Services on his release. Delaying further would have been unjustified based on medical advice and custody time limits (Dilley and Kemp, 2019). This illustrates a difficulty of SMD which, rather than manifesting the danger of violence or self-harm continually, can be episodic, making risk assessment difficult.

Devon Partnership and Devon County Council undertook to learn lessons. G4S Health Services, a UK company providing primary and forensic healthcare services was also involved as employers of Dr Mihal Pichui. They supported Dr Pichui's decision not to conduct a full assessment and stated that he had recommended that the local mental health team saw Lewis-Ranwell the next morning, which recommendation was not acted upon.

Christian Lacey

On 30 March 2018 Christian Lacey's family took him to the Accident and Emergency department of the Royal Liverpool Hospital, UK. Previously he had gone missing in London for several hours, later describing giving a homeless man his new mobile phone because Lacey thought it had been hacked and he was going to die. A mental health worker noted that Lacey 'did not appear to have any mental health issues' (Humphries, 2019).

On 25 April 2018 Lacey unpredictably attacked his father Johan Wierzbick and his half-brother Jacob Carfoot. Lacey entered Carfoot's bedroom holding him in a headlock before Carfoot struggled free and went to a friend's house. Later that evening after his half-brother returned, Lacey held a strangle hold on his father, then punched him before Carfoot intervened (Middleton, 2019). Afraid, the family locked their bedroom doors at night. Carfoot later stated that Lacey believed that the house's bathroom towels were evil (Docking, 2018).

Given the previous day's disturbance, on the morning of 26 April, Lacey was taken to his physician who advised him on anger control techniques. While Lacey was at the surgery, his father found a knife wrapped in clothing in Lacey's bedroom and contacted police. Taken to St Anne Street Police Station, Lacey was assessed by Merseycare staff from the Criminal Justice Liaison Team (Middleton, 2019). They considered that he did not need to be 'sectioned' (legally detained for example in hospital).

Lacey was released on 26 April 2018. Two hours later in the early evening, he stabbed to death his mother Liz aged 63 at her home in Hardy Street, Garston, Liverpool. She was a business adviser for Liverpool Vision. Shortly afterwards, Lacey walked to the nearby home of his 94-year-old grandmother. There he repeatedly stabbed his grandmother's carer Edwina Holden, 54. Rushed to hospital, she survived (Docking, 2018; Middleton, 2019).

Lacey pleaded guilty to the manslaughter of his mother, and to the attempted murder of Edwina Holden (Docking, 2018). Liverpool Crown Court gave Lacey an indefinite hospital order and he was detained at Ashworth Hospital, Merseyside (Humphries, 27 May 2019). Judge Clement

Goldstone ordered Merseycare Foundation Trust to make public a review into what went wrong with Lacey's care (Middleton, 2019).

Gyulchekhra Bobokulova

Born in 1977 in the Samarkand region of Uzbekistan, Gyulchekhra Bobokulova was one of six daughters (Maynaya, 2016). She married three times. She and her first husband Radmir with whom she had three sons, divorced in 2002. Around that time, she was treated for mental illness at a clinic in Uzbekistan and according to her father Bahretdin Turaev imagined voices, became aggressive and lost her memory of some events (Maynaya, 2016). Her second marriage to Sohrob Muminov lasted two years before the couple divorced. In 2014, Bobokulova married Mamour Dzhurakulov (Maynaya, 2016).

While Dzhurakulov remained in Uzbekistan, Bobokulova worked in Moscow as a nanny. In 2012, she was employed by Vladimir and Ekaterina Meshcheryakova. Having been recommended by a family for whom she had previously worked, Bobokulova looked after the Meshcheryakova's younger daughter Anastasia who had developmental disabilities (newsru.com, 2017).

In late 2015, Bobokulova returned to Uzbekistan for a vacation and to renew her passport. She found that her husband had taken a new wife and he offered Bobokulova a secondary role (newsru.com, 2017). Bobokulova, now 38, legally re-entered the Russian Federation at the end of January 2016 and registered with the Federal Immigration Service (TASS, 2016).

Although without a work permit, Bobokulova continued work as a nanny. On the morning of 29 February 2016, she was alone with four-year-old Anastasia after the parents went out with their eldest child. Their apartment occupied the fifth floor of a ten-story residential block on People's Militia Street, Moscow (TASS, 2016). Bobokulova apparently strangled Anastasia (riafan.ru, 2016) before decapitating her with a knife and igniting the apartment. She left the building carrying Anastasia's severed head in a bag (Reporter, 27 April 2016). At 9.30 am the blaze was reported and the fire service shortly arrived, finding the headless body of a child in the apartment (TASS, 2016).

Bobokulova was later seen at the entrance hall of Oktabrskoye Pole Metro Station, North West Moscow holding the decapitated head and threatening to trigger an explosion (In fact, no explosives were found) (TASS, 2016).

Passers-by captured and circulated online mobile phone recordings of Bobokulova shouting 'I am a terrorist' and 'Allahu Akbar'. When police arrived, she told them that she was acting on Allah's orders, and that voices had prompted her to kill Anastasia (Reporter, 27 April 2016). Police detained Bobokulova near the metro at 2.30 pm (newsru.com, 2017).

Bobokulova was arrested on a charge of murdering a minor. Terrorism was initially considered as a motive as the nanny claimed that she was a terrorist when detained (Reporter, 4 March 2016). Bobokulova stated that she killed the girl prompted by online videos of beheadings and by inner voices.

Reportedly, Bobokulova said that she had been driven by hatred, but that she felt sorry for Anastasia, whom she described as 'good' (Reporter, 11 March 2016). In March 2016, the nanny, diagnosed with schizophrenia at the Serbsky Centre, was transferred to a secure psychiatric facility at the Butyrskaya prison, Moscow.

Authorities proposed preventive measures, highlighting the risks of employing an undocumented worker. Pavel Astakhov, Presidential Commissioner for Children's Rights, noted that previously where nannies had harmed children, they usually lacked the required documents or an appropriate contract, and did not understand their responsibilities. He stated that parents hiring a nanny should request a medical examination, and a certificate from a psychiatrist evaluating their mental state (TASS, 2016). Inna Svyatenko, Chairperson of the Moscow City Duma's Commission on Security, cautioned that personnel hired for childcare should have a full medical examination, including a drugs test. She recommended that parents should use proven recruitment agencies and demand letters of recommendation (TASS, 2016).

Timchang Nandap

Timchang Nandap, a Nigerian student seemingly attending London's School of Oriental and African Studies lived in Woolwich, London, and was diagnosed with schizophrenia including delusions of persecution (Davies, 2018a). He experienced hallucinations and had believed that he was a Messiah telepathically able to communicate with others (Evans, 2018). In May 2015, Nandap then aged 23 was seen acting strangely and brandishing a knife on the London street where his sister Wupya lived. Witnesses called police and Nandap was arrested by PC Adam Wellings after a violent struggle (Davies, 2018a).

Having no previous convictions, Nandap was placed on provisional bail. He then flew to Nigeria to visit his family and received clinic treatment for psychosis and anxiety. Returning to the UK in October 2015 he was arrested at Heathrow, charged with the May incident, and bailed for trial. However, the crown prosecutor determined that the evidence was too weak for a successful prosecution and the charge was officially dropped on 23 December 2015 (Davies, 2018a).

Nandap was fatefully to encounter his victim days later. Dutch water engineer Dr Jeroen Ensink, 41, lived in Islington, London and was a senior lecturer in environmental health at the London School of Hygiene and Tropical Medicine (BBC News, 2018; Davies, 2018a). In mid-December 2015, his wife, Nadja Ensink-Teich, a Dutch project manager, gave birth to a daughter, Fleur (Evans, 2018). On 29 December Dr Ensink left his flat to mail birth announcement cards. Nandap, a stranger to Ensink, approached and fatally stabbed him.

An off-duty special constable, Maria Hegarty, who lived nearby heard cries for help. Going to investigate, she found Nandap holding a knife and standing over the victim. Nandap appeared calm but did not respond to her and she attempted CPR (Evans, 2018). Ensink was pronounced dead at the scene about 2.30 pm. (Baker, 2018). Nandap, bare-footed and with blood-stained hands, was later arrested on Camden Road by police officers (Baker, 2018).

Appearing at the Old Bailey, Nandap admitted manslaughter on the grounds of diminished responsibility (BBC News, 2018). It appeared that during the attack he was in a state of cannabis induced psychosis. In October 2016, Nandap was given an indefinite hospital order and held at Broadmoor secure hospital, Berkshire (Evans, 2018).

An inquest into Ensink's death was held in July 2018 at St Pancras Coroner's Court before coroner Mary Hassell (Davies, 2018b). Nandap's older sister, corporate lawyer Wupya Nandap, stated that she had telephoned police in May 2015 raising concerns about his earlier behaviour. Nandap was to be questioned concerning charges of assaulting a police officer and possessing a knife. Wupya told police that her brother had been smoking cannabis and had been watching conspiracy theories on television, both worsening his condition. She warned that he seemed to be experiencing 'paranoia', hallucinations, anxiety, and depression (BBC News, 2018; Davies, 2018a).

Arresting officers, noticing Nandap's strange behaviour had considered the possibility of drug abuse or mental illness. A doctor examined Nandap before the interview and stated that he had been given no 'information' or 'markers' on Nandap's mental health. This was seemingly because another officer had missed information on the custody record. Nandap answered strangely when interviewed. A 'Merlin report' was not created (Davies, 2018a). This report is part of a system used by London's Metropolitan Police Service which can point up vulnerable adults to police officers, social workers, health workers, and staff of other agencies (London Assembly, 2018). In this respect it can assist treatment and prevention.

Geralt Evans, a deputy chief prosecutor at the Crown Prosecution Service, reviewing the case stated that the original decision not to prosecute Nandap for the May incident was 'incorrect'. However, proceeding with a prosecution would not have prevented Nandap from being at liberty to be outside Dr Ensink's home on the day of the killing (Davies, 2018a).

Situational Crime Prevention (SCP)

In an earlier chapter, SCP is fully described and discussed. Briefly, five general strategies are each associated with five opportunity reducing techniques. Regarding the strategy **increase the effort** of perpetrators are the strategies 'target harden', 'control access to facilities', 'screen exits', 'deflect offenders', and 'control tools/weapons'. **Increase the risks** concerns 'extend guardianship', 'assist natural surveillance', 'reduce anonymity', 'utilise place managers', and 'strengthen formal surveillance'. For **reduce rewards** to the perpetrator the techniques are 'conceal targets', 'remove targets', 'identify property', 'disrupt markets', and 'deny benefits'. Regarding **reduce provocations**, techniques comprise 'reduce frustrations and stress', 'avoid disputes', 'reduce emotional arousal', 'neutralise peer pressure', and 'discourage imitation'. **Remove excuses** concerns 'set rules', 'post instructions', 'alert conscience', 'assist compliance', and 'control drugs and alcohol'.

SCP analyses of the four cases

Increasing the effort required of the perpetrator

It was not possible to protect **Lewis-Ranwell's** elderly victims as *targets*. He deludedly believed that all three men participated in child abuse, but his exact targets emerging opportunistically as he scoured Exeter were unpredictable. It was not possible to *control access to facilities* and *screen exits* regarding the specific victims' homes or *deflect the offender* because no crime was anticipated. Opportunity to *control weapons* was lacking because Lewis-Randall killed with everyday tools.

Accordingly, earlier preventive intervention was needed. Key events included Lewis-Ranwell's arrest for disturbance at a local farm, his reluctance to have a mental health assessment, concerns expressed by his mother and a police inspector, threats to farmer Ellis, the medical examiner's view that Lewis-Ranwell was not 'acutely unwell' but would be seen by members of the mental health team, and the lack of a full mental health assessment. Cumulatively, these circumstances suggest an increased risk of violence, but no one saw and evaluated the whole picture or took steps leading to coordinated intervention.

Lacey evaded *control of tools/weapons* because he killed with an easily available knife.

His *targets* were not random but were family members and a carer who was attacked at a family member's home. While this narrowed the range of likely victims, they could not all have been individually protected. The strongest protection to potential victims would have been Lacey being hospitalised for psychiatric care, effectively denying him access to family targets.

Risk indicators suggesting that treatment might be needed included the seeming psychotic episode when Lacey absented himself in London; the attack on his father and half-brother; and Lacey's hiding a knife in his bedroom. All these preceded the killing of his mother and the stabbing of carer Edwina Holden. Furthermore, a review investigating the circumstances indicated procedural and training gaps that hindered Lacey being identified for treatment. Mental health workers did not recognise or diagnose Lacey's untypical schizophrenia with delusions of persecution or explore why he attacked his father and half-brother.

Some members of the Criminal Justice Liaison Team had not received formal training in mental health before joining the team. Police, a physician, and mental health workers may have assumed that Lacey was not dangerous because he was 'well dressed and from a nice family'. Lacey's complex presentation was not 'explored by the practitioners in depth' (Humphries, 2019). Merseycare subsequently ordered new training in recognising psychosis and in assessing risks and issued reminders to staff to properly question the family and carers of mental health patients (Middleton, 2019).

Although in the past, **Bobokulova**'s credentials might have preventively been more fully checked, in the immediate situation leading to Anastasia's death the child was not *hardened as a target* because her parents had left her in the nanny's care. Opportunity to *control access* to the apartment was similarly circumvented. *Screening exits* to the apartment was redundant because Bobokulova had already killed the child before leaving. She was unaffected by *controls applied to weapons* because she killed Anastasia by strangulation.

Accordingly, prevention needed to take place earlier. Bobokulova had been recommended and had worked satisfactorily with the family for three years, so that parents would, in the absence of Bobokulova behaving oddly, have no reason to recognise any risk of violence. Yet Bobokulova had previously been treated for schizophrenia, manifesting as imagined voices, aggression, and lost memories, which may have been exacerbated by marital stress and divorce. In her time working in Moscow, Bobokulova had recently returned from a trip home, discovering that her third husband had demoted her. Wider preventive measures could have involved stricter controls for people working with children such as a register of qualified workers, background checks, up to date references, and perhaps periodic medical and psychological assessments.

With **Nandap**, *hardening the target* Jeroen Ensink was not feasible because Ensinck was killed randomly. *Controlling access* or *screening exits* to the street in Islington where Ensink lived was impracticable because no attack was anticipated. A local special constable attempted to *deflect the offender* but was unable to save Ensink's life. Because Nandap was at liberty, it was not possible to *control the weapon* that he used (a knife).

Probably the most effective way to increase the effort needed for Nandap to harm anyone would have been to remove him from the community into psychiatric care. Risk indicators included Nandap's bizarre behaviour in May when he struggled with a police officer and wielded a knife; the arresting officers' observations of Nandap's strange behaviour and suspicion of drug abuse or mental illness; Wupya Nandap's concerns about her brother's mental state; Nandap's clinic treatment in Nigeria; and his strange responses during a later police interview. Procedurally, better use of the custody record could have been made and fuller information passed to the examining physician. A Merlin report could have been created, highlighting mental health concerns to appropriate personnel in other agencies.

Increasing the risks to the perpetrator

Regarding **Lewis-Ranwell**, opportunities to *extend guardianship* or increase *natural or formal surveillance* prior to the killings were missed or ineffective. A potentially preventive step of his transfer to a Barnstaple homeless centre was negated as Lewis-Ranwell left after threatening to kill a staff member. Once he was free to roam Exeter, residents did not know that he would attack, where he would strike, or whom he would target.

With **Lacey** effective action to *extend guardianship* or improve *natural surveillance* and *formal surveillance* was not taken despite red flags of his strange behaviour in London, and the attacks on his father and half-brother which preceded Lacey killing his mother.

If **Bobokulova** had been recruited through an agency, *extending guardianship* might have been more comprehensive. A check of her credentials and background could have revealed her previous 2002 clinic treatment for schizophrenia, raising questions about her suitability for unsupervised childcare. Because of the nanny's trusted position, *natural surveillance* and *formal surveillance* was limited. *Utilising place managers* such as fitting a supervisory device ('nanny cam') in the apartment, would not have prevented the killing.

Nandap's sister Wupya acted as a whistle blower in carrying out *natural surveillance* but authorities gave insufficient weight to her worries. *Formal surveillance* included the arresting officers' concerns about Nandap's strange behaviour, but these were seemingly not passed to the examining physician. Relatedly, opportunities to *extend guardianship* were missed.

Reducing rewards to the perpetrator

Lewis-Ranwell's 'reward' was his deluded belief that he was saving previously abused children, requiring psychiatric treatment to deal with the delusions. Lewis-Ranwell's victims could effectively have been *concealed* or *removed as targets* by admitting him to psychiatric care before the fatal attacks.

With **Lacey**, there were no rewards to reduce because his attacks were perpetrated for no 'reason' that he could provide. *Concealing* or *removing targets* (Lacey's earlier family targets, his mother, and his grandmother's carer) could have been achieved by admitting him to psychiatric care.

Bobokulova's actions may have led to deluded psychological 'rewards' relating to her belief that she was complying with Allah's guidance. However, she gained no real-life benefits from killing. Anastasia was not *concealed* or *removed* as a *target* because her parents saw no risk.

With **Nandap**, there were no rewards to reduce because he killed randomly and irrationally. *Concealing* or *removing targets* in the sense of Nandap's then unknown victim would have required removing Nandap to psychiatric care. Once Nandap was at liberty it was impossible to *conceal* or *remove* Ensink as a target because Nandap's subsequent actions were unknown.

Reducing provocations towards the perpetrator

No techniques to reduce provocations applied to **Lewis-Ranwell** whose attacks stemmed from false beliefs rather than from reducible *frustrations and stress*, avoidable *disputes*, or neutralizable *peer pressure*. Any source or emotional context of Lewis-Randall's false beliefs about child abuse and torture are unknown. Consequently, one cannot know whether in the longer-term *reducing emotional arousal* might have been preventive.

Avoiding disputes or *reducing frustrations and stress* or *reducing emotional arousal* seem inapplicable in the relationships between **Lacey**, his father, and half-brother. There is no evidence of his being in a real-life dispute, or of the victims frustrating or emotionally arousing Lacey at the time.

Bobokulova claimed that driven by hatred, she was prompted to kill by online videos of beheadings and by inner voices. Her actions may have partly related to marital *frustrations and stress* so that efforts to *reduce* these may have been preventive. If Bobokulova had not had access to online depictions of beheadings this could have closed one avenue of potential influence and avoided encouraging *imitation*.

It is unclear to what extent **Nandap's** psychotic episodes were influenced by reducible *frustrations and stress* or *emotional arousal*. His sister reported that he watched television programmes about conspiracy theories and smoked cannabis, exacerbating his disturbed state. There was no *dispute* to *avoid* between Nandap and Ensink because the killing was (to all outside observation) unprovoked.

Removing perpetrators' excuses

Lacey did not try to justify his actions. **Lewis-Ranwell** did not seek excuses to kill that required removing, because he believed that he was acting morally. **Bobokulova** was convinced that she was instructed by Allah. *Controlling drugs and alcohol* might have been preventive with Bobokulova as some (unconfirmed) reports mention her appearing intoxicated. **Nandap's** sister considered that his cannabis use worsened his condition.

Overview of preventive issues

Recognising and acting on indications of increased risk of violence

A series of risk indicators were apparent, particularly for Lewis-Ranwell, Lacey, and Nandap. For example, with **Lewis-Ranwell** these included arrest for disturbance at a local farm, his reluctance to have a mental health assessment, concerns expressed by his mother and later by a police inspector, and Lewis-Ranwell's threats to farmer Ellis. Cumulatively, these circumstances suggested increased risk of violence.

With **Lacey,** there was the seeming psychotic episode during Lacey's absence in London; the attack on his father and half-brother; and Lacey's hiding a knife in his bedroom, all preceding the killing of his mother and the stabbing of Edwina Holden.

Nandap exhibited bizarre behaviour in May, struggling with a police officer and wielding a knife. Arresting officers observing his strange behaviour suspected drug abuse or mental illness. Wupya Nandap expressed concerns about her brother's deteriorating mental state. Nandap required treatment in Nigeria and responded strangely during his later interview. Such concerns it appears were insufficiently conveyed to the physician who examined Nandap.

In these instances, there was evidence of accumulating risk of violence that seemingly was not sufficiently recognised. But still left open is the question of which person or agency would act and what action could they take. One scenario is that a mental health professional gains information from their own investigations and from other agencies to initiate taking an individual into psychiatric care for their own safety and/or the safety of others.

Correctly assessing and evaluating SMD

The nature of SMD can make its assessment complex as with episodic features of some aspects of schizophrenia. *DSM-5* (American Psychiatric Association, 2013), describing the development and course of schizophrenia, mentions that, 'many remain chronically ill, with exacerbations and remissions of active symptoms' (Ibid., p. 102). Diagnostic 'specifiers' of the course of extended schizophrenia include 'multiple episodes' which involve at least 'a first episode, a remission and a minimum of one relapse'. Multiple episodes can present themselves as an 'acute episode', 'partial remission', and 'full remission' (Ibid., p. 100).

A forensic medical examiner saw **Lewis-Ranwell** in his detention cell and evaluated him to be not 'acutely unwell', and a full mental health assessment was not ordered. However, given the context of Lewis-Ranwell's previous behaviour (of which the physician was apparently not apprised), such absence of acute illness may have been a phase in a pattern of recurring episodes of illness and relative wellness.

A condition's complex presentation and the general appearance of an individual can complicate assessment. A review found that **Lacey's** behaviour when examined by mental health professionals was untypical of schizophrenia with delusions of persecution. A mental health worker seemingly noted that Lacey was a 'pleasant young man' who 'did not appear to have any mental health issues'. When Lacey was taken to St Anne Street Police Station and assessed by Merseycare staff from the Criminal Justice Liaison Team he was judged not to require admission to psychiatric care. The review also suggested that police, a general practitioner, and mental health workers may have assumed that Lacey was not dangerous because of his appearance and background. Lacey's complex presentation was not explored in enough depth.

The role of psychiatric care as protection and prevention

Clearly, some individual victims could not have been protected from the random or spontaneous attacks of someone experiencing severe mental disorder. This can be because there was no suspicion that they might be harmed as with Anastasia in

Bobokulova's care. Or there may be indications of the risk of potential harm to family members and others but perhaps too many to arrange individual protection as with Lacey. There may be concerns more generally, although specific victims cannot be predicted as with Nandap and with Lewis-Randall.

In these instances, protecting possible victims and society generally would involve removing of the potential perpetrator to psychiatric care, physically preventing access to potential victims in the community. This also enables treating harmful delusions such as Lewis-Randall's fixed belief that he was rescuing children.

This raises challenges. As well as being precise about who will decide to admit a person to psychiatric care, including involuntarily, it needs to be clear what type of evidence will normally be necessary. This implies that evidence is pooled and conveyed clearly and in a timely way to decision makers. In the longer term it involves an evaluation of the decisions made and how effective and appropriate they were. Similar issues arise in relation to the use of agencies and better supervision of workers with children as discussed later.

Improving communications among professionals

Clarity about professional roles and expectations and, relatedly, clear lines of communication are important to ensure effective interventions. The medical examiner's judgement that **Lewis-Ranwell** was not 'acutely unwell' was conveyed. But his expectation that the detainee would be seen by members of the mental health team, seems not to have been communicated clearly to someone with the authority to ensure such an assessment was carried out. If such an intention was conveyed, it was not followed through. Whatever the intentions or expectations, no full mental health assessment was made.

Communication between police and medical professionals was not clear enough regarding **Nandap**. Arresting officers had noticed his behaving strangely and wondered if it was owing to drug abuse or mental illness. A doctor examining Nandap before his interview with police claimed that he had been given no 'markers' on his mental health, apparently because another officer had missed the information on the custody record.

Improving training and procedural understanding

A review investigating the **Lacey** case indicated procedural and training issues that hindered Lacey's condition being identified and treated. Mental health workers did not diagnose Lacey's behaviour as schizophrenia with delusions of persecution because it was untypical. Neither did they explore why he had attacked his father and half-brother. Some Criminal Justice Liaison Team members had not received formal training in mental health before joining the group. Various professionals may have been misled because of Lacey's appearance and family background. Among recommendations therefore was new training in recognising psychosis and in assessing risks, and reminders to properly question the family and carers of mental health patients.

With **Nandap,** procedurally, better use of the custody record could have been made and fuller information passed to the examining physician. Crucially a Merlin report could have been created highlighting mental health concerns to others.

The use of agencies and better supervision of workers with children

Bobokulova had been recommended and had worked without problems with Anastasia's family for three years. However, it seems they were unaware of the nanny's 2002 clinic treatment for schizophrenia, possibly exacerbated by marital stresses and divorce. An unrecognised trigger for her returning schizophrenia therefore may have been Bobokulova's discovery that her third husband had demoted her as a marriage partner. This points to stricter controls for workers with children including using agencies, a register of qualified personnel, background checks, and up to date references. Suggested periodic medical and psychological assessments would involve considerable resources and administration.

Where there is a perceived safety risk, it must be clear what type and level of evidence will be sufficient to disbar a person from working with children (or other vulnerable people). In the longer term, authorities should establish what evidence will be available to show that the approach is successfully protecting children.

Controlling the abuse of drugs and internet content

Tighter control of skunk cannabis, might have prevented Nandap's access to it, reducing his drive to harm others. However, such control where individuals are intent on obtaining drugs is difficult. **Bobokulova** may have been influenced by internet images of beheadings, whose stricter control may have been preventive. Again, the practicalities of achieving such control are challenging.

Practical situational approaches

Published problem-specific guides cover various issues and provide evidence for their working (Arizona State University Center for Problem Oriented Policing, various dates). They include guidance and evidence relating to people with mental disorders as offenders and victims (Cordner, 2006). Approaches involve analysing local issues to better understand contributory factors, establishing a baseline for measuring effectiveness, and reviewing responses to the problems. While aimed at the police, the guidance indicates a multi service and community response.

Among approaches to *improve police response to incidents* are 'training generalist police officers' to deal with problems involving people with SMD. 'Providing more information to patrol officers' relates to information about support facilities in the community to which individuals could be referred and (within protection of privacy limits) making available information about community members with mental disorders. 'Deploying specialist police officers' refers to having generalist police officers with specialist training who could also be deployed in situations involving individuals with SMD. Another strategy is 'deploying specialised non police responders'.

Working with stakeholders includes 'initiating assisted outpatient treatment' which involves legal enforcement of treatment plans, for example taking prescribed medication. 'Establishing crisis response sites' concerns facilities (usually in a hospital) to which police can transport individuals with SMD. They provide streamlined intake procedures and have a 'no-refusal' policy to police, guaranteeing that the individual will at least be evaluated. 'Establishing jail-based diversion' involves special procedures channelling an offender with SMD to treatment rather than jail when the case is reviewed for prosecution, or when it comes to court.

Turning to *targeting offenders*, this involves 'targeting repeat criminals' with mental disorders by using involuntary commitment to psychiatric care, better guardianship, court-ordered medication, or restraining orders. In 'targeting those responsible for repeat or chronic disturbances' who have mental disorder, police have used criminal charges and probation conditions to control a person's disruptive behaviour, while empowering the community to better supervise the behaviour.

Targeting locations has implicated 'regulating facilities more effectively'. Police in Lancashire, UK noticed that certain mental health facilities had higher rates of people going missing and walking away. This implicated management practices, and the physical features of security of facilities. The constabulary appointed liaison officers to enable venues to improve security and practices, then negotiated performance targets for each facility. Subsequently, if a venue exceeds its annual missing persons limit, it comes under government review, risking losing its license and funding.

Conclusion

Situational Crime Prevention was used to analyse four cases of homicide by individuals with SMD. Regarding **increasing the effort required of the perpetrator** strategies, such as protecting the victims as targets, were largely impracticable. In the four instances, better prevention would likely have included psychiatric care. Often, accumulating signs of risk of violence were not seen holistically because of limitations in communication procedures and database systems.

Turning to **increasing the risks to the perpetrator**, risk indicators were sometimes not followed through. In Nandap's case, authorities gave insufficient weight to his sister's warnings, and the arresting officers' concerns about Nandap's strange behaviour were not passed to the examining physician.

Regarding **reducing rewards to the perpetrator**, victims could have been effectively *concealed* or *removed as targets* by admitting Lewis-Ranwell, Lacey, and Nandap to psychiatric care before their fatal attacks.

Concerning **reducing provocations towards the perpetrator**, the actions of Bobokulova may have been partly related to marital *frustrations and stress*. Efforts to *reduce* these had they been known, for example through counselling and support, may have been preventive. Stopping her accessing online depictions of beheadings could have avoided her desire to imitate it, if not through technological prevention, then indirectly through counselling and support

Concerning **removing perpetrators' excuses**, neither Lewis-Ranwell nor Bobokulova sought to excuse their actions because they were experiencing delusions at the time of the killings. Nandap's sister believed his cannabis use worsened his condition.

Various preventive issues emerged from the SCP analyses.

Recognising and acting on indications of increased risk of violence

Risk indicators were apparent, particularly for Lewis-Ranwell, Lacey, and Nandap, which were not always seen holistically enough to lead to intervention. With **Lewis-Ranwell**, for example, cumulative circumstances indicated increased risk of violence.

Correctly assessing and evaluating severe mental disorder

The nature of severe mental disorder can make its assessment complex, leading to indications being missed. Episodic features of some forms and manifestations of schizophrenia are an example, as suggested by the cases of Lewis-Ranwell, and of Lacey.

The role of psychiatric care as protection and prevention

Sometimes potential victims cannot be individually protected. This can be because there was no suspicion that they might be harmed, or there may too many potential victims to make individual protection practicable, or specific victims cannot be predicted. Here, protecting potential victims would likely involve removing of the potential perpetrator to psychiatric care, physically preventing access to potential victims, and enabling treatment.

Improving communications among professionals

Clarity about professional roles and expectations and clear lines of communication facilitate effective interventions. Communication between police and medical professionals are not always clear enough.

Improving training and understanding of procedures

Mental health workers can miss untypical presentations of severe mental disorder or insufficiently enquire into circumstances. This necessitates retraining in recognising psychosis and in assessing risks, and reminders to properly question the family and carers of mental health patients. Sometimes the custody record needs to be used better and fuller information passed to the examining physician. Overarching reports alerting various agencies are sometimes not made.

The use of agencies and better supervision of workers with children

Stricter controls for people working with children could include the wider use of agencies for qualified workers rather than informal direct employment by parents, a register of qualified workers, background checks, up to date references, and possibly periodic medical and psychological assessments.

Controlling the abuse of drugs and internet content

The cases considered suggest tighter control of skunk cannabis, and violent internet videos such as beheadings, although both are challenging.

Practical situation-based approaches

Examples of interventions involving police and others aim to fill cracks in provision or services, liaison, and communication. If not addressed, these can precipitate increased risks to people with severe mental disorder, leading to greater risks of violence. This approach has included improving police response to incidents, working with stakeholders, targeting offenders, and targeting locations.

Suggested activities

Read the guidance and evidence including US and UK examples in the document by Cordner (2006) *People with Mental Illness* www.popcenter.asu.edu/con tent/people-mental-illness. Select several interventions and reconfigure them as guidance in which a service other than police will initiate the action. This could be health services, hospitals, clinics, the prison system, and the probation service.

Key texts

Ewing, C. P. (2008) *Insanity: Murder, Madness and the Law.* Oxford, Oxford University Press.

This book presents ten examples of homicides which, while controversial, indicate how contemporary use is made of the insanity defence and the complex issues arising.

References

American Psychiatric Association (2013) *Diagnostic and Statistical Manual of Mental Disorders Fifth Edition (DSM-5)*. Washington DC, APA.

Arizona State University Center for Problem Oriented Policing (various dates). https://popcenter.asu.edu/.

Baker, K. (2018) 'Why was mentally ill man set free to kill my husband?' *Mail Online* (2 July 2018) www.dailymail.co.uk/news/article-5909435/ Psychotic-killer-stabbed-renowned-academic-death-outside-home.html.

BBC News (2018) 'Jeroen Ensink inquest: Killer's sister had warned police' BBC News (3 July 2018) www.bbc.co.uk/news/uk-england-london-44693781.

Cordner, G. (2006) *People with Mental Illness* (Guide No. 40) Arizona State University Center for Problem Oriented Policing. https://popcenter.asu.edu/content/people-mental-illness.

Davies, C. (2018a) '"They're coming to get me": Troubled student who killed an academic' *The Guardian* (17 July 2018) www.theguardian.com/uk-news/2018/jul/17/femi-nandap-troubled-student-killed-academic.

Davies, C. (2018b) 'Inquest criticises police over London killing of Dutch academic' *The Guardian* (17 July 2018) www.theguardian.com/uk-news/2018/jul/17/inquest-criticises-police-over-london-killing-of-dutch-academic-jeroen-ensink.

Dilley, S. and Kemp, P. (2019) 'Alexander Lewis-Ranwell: The triple killer who was arrested twice' BBC News (2 December 2019) www.bbc.co.uk/news/uk-england-devon-50591491.

Docking, N. (2018) 'Man stabbed his mum to death and tried to kill his gran's carer in psychotic episode' *Echo* (21 December 2018) www.liverpoolecho.co.uk/ news/liverpool-news/christian-lacey-liz-lacey-murder-15584632.

Evans, M. (2018) 'Widow of academic stabbed to death on his doorstep demands to know why psychotic knifeman was released to kill' *Telegraph* (2 July 2018) www.telegraph.co.uk/ news/2018/07/02/psychotic-killer-attacked-new-father-told-police-leave-dead/.

Humphries, J. (2019) 'Son's brutal killing of mum could have been avoided if not for "deadly errors"' *Mirror* (27 May 2019) www.mirror.co.uk/news/uk-news/sons-brutal-killing-mum-could-16208553.

London Assembly (2018) 'Merlin CAN Reports' (19 July 2018) www.london.gov.uk/ questions/ 2018/1733.

Maynaya, E. (2016) 'She repeated to me, "I am afraid dad"' *Gazeta.ru* (3 February 2016) www.gazeta.ru/politics/2016/03/02_a_8105087.shtml.

Middleton, J. (2019) 'Too middle class to kill: Son with schizophrenia was left to stab his mother to death as doctors and police thought he was too well-healed to be dangerous' *Mail Online* (27 May 2019) www.dailymail.co.uk/news/article-7074549/Police-medics-missed-two-chances-stop-mentally-ill-man-killing-mother-report-finds.html.

Morris, S. (2019) 'Killer of three elderly Devon men found not guilty of murder due to insanity' *The Guardian* (2 December 2019) www.theguardian.com/uk-news/2019/dec/02/killer-of-three-elderly-devon-men-found-not-guilty-due-to-insanity.

newsru.com (2017) 'Police detain a woman with a child's severed head near Moscow metro' newsru.com (29 February 2016, updated 6 December 2017) (in Russian) www.newsru.com/russia/29feb2016/oktpole.html.

Reporter (11 March 2016) 'Moscow nanny says 'voices' told her to commit murder' *The Moscow Times* (11 March 2016) www.themoscowtimes.com/2016/03/11/moscow-nanny-says-voices-told-her-to-commit-murder-a52134.

Reporter (4 March 2016) 'Nanny charged with murder of 4-year old child in Moscow' *The Moscow Times* (4 March 2016) www.themoscowtimes.com/2016/03/04/nanny-charged-with-murder-of-4-year-old-child-in-moscow-a52076.

Reporter (27 April 2016) 'Moscow nanny charged with beheading child sent to psychiatric prison' *The Moscow Times* (27 April 2016) www.themoscowtimes.com/2016/04/27/moscow-nanny-charged-with-beheading-child-sent-to-psychiatric-prison-a52700.

riafan.ru (2016) 'Killer nanny strangled the girl before cutting off her head' riafan.ru (29 February 2016) https://riafan.ru/506049-nyanya-ubiica-zadushila-devochku-pered-tem-kak-otrezat-ei-golovu.

Sky News (2019) 'Paranoid schizophrenic Alexander Lewis-Ranwell not guilty of murdering three pensioners' Sky News (2 December 2019) https://news.sky.com/story/paranoid-schizophrenic-man-not-guilty-of-murderers-three-pensioners-hours-apart-11876554.

TASS (2016) 'The murder of a child in Moscow: Investigation progress and public reaction' TASS (29 February 2016) https://tass.ru/proisshestviya/2706157.

Chapter 7

Means, motive, opportunity, location

Introduction

Aspects of crime featuring in the Situational Crime Prevention model (Clarke, 2018) include weapons used in committing an offence, the opportunity structure supporting a crime, and the environment in which it takes place. Relating to these are respectively means, opportunity, and location. Motive is less evident in SCP, but its behavioural expressions can arguably be inferred. Means, motive, opportunity, and location are relevant to crime in general, and to homicide including that perpetrated by individuals with severe mental disorder (SMD).

In the ensuing sections, cases are cited, with an illustrative reference at their first mention. Fuller details of these cases and further references are included in the book's glossary.

Situational Crime Prevention (SCP)

SCP, fully described in an earlier chapter, proposes five general strategies each associated with five opportunity reducing techniques. Regarding the strategy *increase the effort* of perpetrators are the strategies 'target harden', 'control access to facilities', 'screen exits', 'deflect offenders', and 'control tools/weapons'. *Increase the risks* concerns 'extend guardianship', 'assist natural surveillance', 'reduce anonymity', 'utilise place managers', and 'strengthen formal surveillance'. For *reduce rewards* to the perpetrator the techniques are 'conceal targets', 'remove targets', 'identify property', 'disrupt markets', and 'deny benefits'. Regarding *reduce provocations*, techniques comprise 'reduce frustrations and stress', 'avoid disputes', 'reduce emotional arousal', 'neutralise peer pressure', and 'discourage imitation'. *Remove excuses* concerns 'set rules', 'post instructions', 'alert conscience', 'assist compliance', and 'control drugs and alcohol'.

Means of killing

'Means' in the present context is a method, or a path of action, or an instrument used to achieve a certain end, or to accomplish something. With

DOI: 10.4324/9781003172727-9

homicide, the means involves taking actions such as physically attacking or manually strangling or using a tool or weapon.

Homicides by individuals with SMD and homicides generally

Means of killing used by individuals with SMD have included beating or bludgeoning the victim using hands and feet, or with an implement or tool such as a piece of wood or a hammer; firearms and 'edge weapons' such as a knife, a sword, or scissors. A vehicle may be driven at a victim at speed.

For homicides generally, 2018 FBI data on murders in the US categorises 'firearms' (72.7%), 'knives or cutting instruments' (10.7%), 'unknown or other dangerous weapons' (11.8%), and 'personal weapons such as hand fists and feet' (4.8%) (Federal Bureau of Investigation, 2018). Individuals with SMD use similar means although not in the same percentages. Also, means such as poisoning usually requiring detailed planning are less evident with SMD homicides (Farrell, 2017, pp. 131–133). Attempts have been made to relate weapons and motivation. An analysis of data from Newark, New Jersey, suggested that domestically motivated homicides are most likely to be committed with knives and blunt objects. On the other hand, drug-, gang-, dispute-, revenge-, and robbery-motivated homicides were most likely to involve a firearm (Pelletier, 2017).

A review of nine studies of relationships between psychosis and means of homicide found that the great majority of perpetrators with psychosis had been symptomatic at the time of the offence (Minero, Barker and Bedford, 2017). In countries where guns were more available, their use was more common as indicated by a US study which found 48% of their sample of people with SMD incarcerated for murder used guns (Matejkowski, Cullen and Solomon, 2008). In countries where guns were less available, other means were commoner. A study in England and Wales looking at mental illness in people who kill strangers, found that 37% used knives and only 2% used guns (Shaw et al., 2004). Overall, homicide weapons used by people with mental disorder reflect what is available.

Edge weapons

Edge weapons include those having points to stab and blades to cut and slash, for example knives, swords, bayonets, and axes (www.policeone.com) and are the commonest means used in the cases considered in this chapter. The review already mentioned of nine studies of relationships between psychosis and means of homicide found five out of the nine articles showed an association between schizophrenia/delusional disorder and the use of sharp instruments as a method of homicide (Minero, Barker and Bedford, 2017).

A knife was used by Christian Lacey to stab his mother Liz Lacey (Docking, 2018), by Timchang Nandap to kill engineer Jeroen Ensink (Evans, 2018), by Michael Harris to stab his best friend Carl James

(Reporter, 2 August 2007), and by Deyan Devanov to behead Jennifer Mills-Westley (Gilligan, 2013). After fatally stabbing her seven children and a niece, Raina Thaiday stabbed herself repeatedly but not fatally (Australian Associated Press, 2017). Phillip Simelane knifed schoolgirl Christina Edkins in the chest (Welton, 2013). After chasing his former partner Colette Lynch from her house into the street, Percy Wright stabbed her to death (Twomey, 2009). Peter Atkins broke into the house of his son-in-law Stephen Provoost and his wife (Atkins' daughter), killing him with a sheath knife (Savill, 2001). While her husband was at work, Dena Schloser cut off the arms of her baby daughter Margaret (Joyner, 2004). Gregory Davis knifed Dorothy Rogers, a drinking acquaintance, then stabbed and disembowelled her son (BBC News, 2003).

Sometimes more than one knife is used or another bladed weapon. When Ashleigh Ewing, an employee of a mental health charity, visited Ronald Dixon, he stabbed her repeatedly with knives (NHS England, 2013). Nathan Jones killed his mother Pamela Ann Jones at her home seemingly using two knives (Reporter, 18 December 2007). Marc Carter stabbed Gino Nelmes, a fellow resident in a mental health supported housing property, with a Samurai sword (Reporter, 3 April 2006).

Beating and bludgeoning

Beating involves the repeated use of fists and feet. Bludgeoning implies repeated striking with a blunt instrument such as a club. Where a weapon is used, it may be carried to the scene or found in situ. Vitali Davydov killed his psychiatrist Wayne Fenton at the doctor's office by beating him with fists (Barr, Londoño and Morse, 2006). Alexander Lewis-Ranwell attacked one elderly man with a hammer and later killed two more with a spade, finding each item on the victim's premises (Morris, 2019). William Bruce killed his mother with a hatchet as she worked at her desk (Bernstein and Koppel, 2008). Bludgeoning their heads with a rock, Deana Laney killed her young sons (Falkenberg, 2003).

Firearms

Alexander Bonds shot police officer Miosotis Familia in the head at close range with a stolen revolver (Celona and Golding, 2017). Mark Tyler killed his mother with a sawn-off shotgun before two days later shooting himself with the same weapon (BBC, 2013).

Driving a vehicle

Marie Elise West deliberately and repeatedly drove her car over Jesus Plascencia in a car park (Teetor, 2002). University freshman David Attias drove his Saab at speed into a group of young adults, killing four (Lagos, 2002).

Strangulation

Broadly, strangulation involves blood supply to part of the body being cut off (as with a 'strangulated' hernia). In homicides, strangulation usually refers to a perpetrator deliberately preventing blood supply reaching the brain, constricting the victim's neck manually or with a ligature. Nanny Gyulchekhra Bobokulova manually strangled four-year-old Anastasia Meshcheryakova before beheading her (TASS, 2016).

Drowning

Drowning refers to respiratory impairment and stoppage caused by being immersed in a liquid. While her husband was at work, Lisa Ann Diaz, drowned their two young daughters in a bathtub at home believing that she was saving them from a worse fate (Ellis and Emily, 2006). Four out of nine studies considered by Minero, Barker and Bedford (2017) revealed an association between mood disorders (bipolar disorder/major depression) and strangulation, drowning, asphyxiation, or suffocation.

Multiple means of homicide

Using multiple means of killing suggests a prolonged attack. Timothy Crook kicked, punched, and stamped on his elderly parents, hit them with a hammer, and strangled them with a belt (BBC News, 2015). Keith Michael Addy hit escort Annamarie Lewandowski with a hammer and then stabbed her before dismembering her body (Milwaukee County Case 2003CF001468).

Available weapons and weapons taken to the scene

Using available weapons includes hitting a victim with hands and/or feet and manual strangulation. It also involves using everyday items like rocks available in the vicinity (Deana Laney), and tools such as hammer or a spade (Alexander Lewis-Ranwell). A car as an everyday device driven at speed at the victim(s) has been used for killing (Marie Elise West; David Attias).

Knives already on the premises may be used where killing occurs in the perpetrator's home as with Raina Thaiday who stabbed her children and a niece; Dena Schloser who amputated her baby daughter's arms; Ronald Dixon who killed a mental health worker visiting him at home, and Nathan Jones who stabbed his mother at their shared home.

Knives may be either carried by the perpetrator or be known to be available at the scene. A knife was carried by Gregory Davis (to his victims' home), Phillip Simelane (onto a bus), Michael Harris (outside his friend's house), Timchang Nandap (in the street); Percy Wright (to his former partner's dwelling), Deyan Devanov (to a local store) Peter Atkins (to his daughter's and son-in-law's residence), and by Christian Lacey (to his mother's home). Marc Carter used a previously purchased Samurai sword.

Excessive and dramatic violence

In some homicides the level and type of violence is dramatically excessive and sustained, eliciting media clichés such as 'frenzied attack'. Four-year-old Anastasia Meshcheryakova was beheaded by Gyulchekhra Bobokulova. Devanov beheaded grandmother Jennifer Mills-Westley. Schloser severed the arms of Margaret, her baby daughter. Davis stabbed and disembowelled Michael Rogers, and Addy killed and dismembered escort Annamarie Lewandowski.

Stabbing is often described as 'repeated' as when mental health charity worker Ashleigh Ewing was killed by Ronald Dixon. Peter Atkins repeatedly stabbed Stephen Provoost with a sheath knife. Using a Samurai sword, Marc Carter stabbed Gino Nelmes, a fellow supported housing resident, 18 times including through the heart, liver, and spleen.

Multiple means of killing also illustrates excessive violence. Crook killed his parents by kicking, punching, stamping, hitting with a hammer, and strangling. Addy killed escort Annamarie Lewandowski by blows with a hammer and by stabbing.

Means and prevention

Prevention related to the means of homicide includes controlling access to firearms by using background checks, especially for a potential perpetrator with SMD. Police can reduce the number of people carrying offensive edge weapons through 'stop and search' powers. Roadside barriers in busy cities can protect pedestrians from vehicle attack and have been installed following terrorist incidents such as the 2006 truck attack in Nice, France. Such preventive steps are less feasible where homicide does not involve a physical weapon. This applies to 'personal weapons' including beating, manual strangulation, and drowning. It also encompasses bludgeoning which can involve using almost any blunt object, and ligature strangulation which can implicate practically any cord, rope, or belt.

SCP identifies prevention strategies relevant to the means of homicide. These include 'hardening targets' by erecting roadside barriers to protect pedestrians from vehicle attacks, 'controlling tools/weapons' including the sale and use of firearms and edge weapons, 'strengthening formal surveillance', which can apply to police stop and search powers, and 'disrupting markets', which can involve customs officers and others seizing illegally imported firearms.

Motive, psychological/behavioural aspects, homicide, and criminal prosecution

One conceptualisation of motive proposes a 'homicide event motive' focusing on the fundamental reason for the homicide. It takes account of not only the offender's personal reasoning, but also the homicide situation and the elements that brought it about (Parker and McKinley, 2018).

Petri and Cofer (2019) refer to 'forces acting either on or within a person to initiate behaviour'. Motivation is seen as an internal drive which leads a person to behave in a certain way. It is also affected by surroundings as with hunger, a physiological drive, which can be stimulated by the presence of certain types of food. So called primary motives are unlearned and include hunger, sex, and perhaps aggression. Secondary motives are learned, can differ from person to person and may include power and achievement (Ibid.).

Where motive is seen as a driving force behind actions, it may be envisaged as a psychological phenomenon, within a social context. Showing the existence of a motive in a court of law is likely to involve giving examples of a suspected per-petrator's behaviour, suggesting a compelling force. An accused may have expressed hatred either towards the victim or to others either verbally or in writing such as texts, e-mails, or letters; or shown avarice through excessive concern about money. Supposed subjective motivating traits such as avarice can overlap with behavioural and social indicators like financial gain.

Stating a motive for a homicide suggests why the killing took place. Motives may overlap and interact with each other, may be speculative, or can remain unknown. A broad motive for a homicide might be financial gain from life insur-ance, sexual freedom from an unwanted spouse, jealousy, revenge, or sadism. Also, within a homicide, a perpetrator's choices around a killing can raise motive related questions. Why was this location chosen? Why was this type of weapon selected?

With criminal prosecution, it is unnecessary to prove motive. An exception is hate crime when prosecutors must demonstrate that the defendant was moti-vated by hatred towards a victim having protected status. Motive can assume importance when defence lawyers suggest that a defendant had no reason for committing the crime (and the prosecution argue otherwise). It can be important in police investigations attempting to understand why an offence was committed. In sentencing, an offender's motive – base or well-intentioned – can influence a court's decisions about penalties.

Motive and SMD

Voices commanding action (including to save the victim)

Diaz drowned her two young daughters in a bathtub at home, believing that she suffered numerous ailments which she had transmitted to her children. At the time of the killings, she had delusions that evil spirits occupied her home, and voices told her that her daughters would painfully die. She saw supposed omens that she and the girls must die that day while voices in her head told her 'This is the day you have to do it'.

Addy bludgeoned and dismembered escort Annamarie Lewandowski telling detectives that he was directed by voices and possessed by demons. Bobokulova strangled then beheaded four-year-old Anastasia Meshcheryakova, later informing police that Allah had ordered her to act, and that voices had prompted her to kill the girl. In the Spanish Canary Islands Devanov beheaded a retired resident, Jennifer Mills-Westley, believing that he was Jesus Christ sent to create a new Jerusalem and had heard voices commanding him to kill.

Deana Laney beat her young sons' heads with a rock because God 'told her' to kill them. A year earlier, she had informed fellow church members that the world was ending, and God had ordered her to get her house in order. A court judged that she had psychotic delusions at the time of the killing. In Australia, Raina Thaiday killed seven of her children and a niece. Psychiatrists considered that long-term cannabis use triggered schizophrenia and that Thaiday believed that she heard a bird call signalling the end of the world and killed the children to save them.

Animosity towards the victim or a wider group

For 18 years, Peter Atkins had schizophrenia. Over time, he developed animosity towards his son-in-law Stephen Provoost whom he finally stabbed to death. He told police of the killing, 'It did not seem real to me. It was like a dream'. Alexander Bonds had been convicted for assaulting a police officer. His social media posts indicated his hatred of police so his random shooting of officer Miosotis Familia may have been directed at police generally.

Conviction that the victim threatens the perpetrator

The judge in the case of Phillip Simelane who killed schoolgirl Christina Edkins on a public bus concluded that Simelane's mental function was 'wholly abnormal'. This was owing to Simelane's mental disorder and that he killed in a 'deluded state' thinking that the victim endangered him. Marc Carter, while in a supported housing property in England, killed fellow resident Gino Nelmes with a Samurai sword, believing that Nelmes was reading his thoughts and repeating them. Davydov, who had schizophrenia, killed psychiatrist Wayne Fenton who had agreed to see him as an emergency patient. Seemingly, there was an altercation about Davydov taking his medication and after the attack he told police that he feared a sexual assault.

Beliefs antipathetic to the victim

Alexander Lewis-Ranwell falsely believed that his elderly victims were paedophiles. Anthony Paine, he thought, was holding a kidnapped girl in his cellar, and Dick and Roger Carter he believed to have perpetrated child abuse and torture. He presumably aimed to rescue the 'victims' and to punish the supposed offenders. William Bruce killed his mother Amy believing that she was an al Qaeda agent.

General feelings of persecution and threat

Lacey, in killing his mother and later non-fatally stabbing his grandmother's carer, may have been influenced by feelings of threat and persecution. However, the nature of the threat and how it reposed in the victims were unclear. Crook who killed his elderly parents Robert and Elsie, at some point believed that police were conspiring against him and US forces were pursuing him. Again, the exact motive for killing his parents remains unknown.

Mission to kill

Davis, who killed Dorothy Rogers and her son Michael, aspired to become a serial killer and kept a diary recoding his plans and hopes to kill worldwide. Student David Attias drove his Saab at speed into a group of young adults, killing four of them, then climbed on top of his vehicle declaring that he was, 'the angel of death'.

Unclear motive (including possibly drug related)

Marie Elise West was repeatedly arrested and hospitalised over many years after being diagnosed with bipolar disorder. She had previously claimed that she was the Messiah and warned elementary school students against being sold as sex slaves. On the evening of the killing, believing that Michael Maglieri, a club owner's son, would be killed, she drove to 'rescue' him. In a parking lot she repeatedly ran over Latina Jesus Plascencia in her vehicle. It is unclear if this related to West's original 'rescue' notion. Found 'Not guilty' of a racial hate crime but guilty of second-degree murder, she was later judged insane.

Dixon, who experienced schizophrenia with delusions of persecution, stabbed mental health charity worker, Ashleigh Ewing, seemingly resenting her delivering a letter about debts he owed the charity. Nathan Jones, living with his mother, stabbed her after acting increasingly psychotically that day. Having a history of postpartum depression and seemingly during a psychotic episode, Schloser severed her baby daughter's arms. Wright stabbed his former partner Colette Lynch after his mental health had deteriorated over an extended period.

Tyler was known to police, probation, mental health, and drug support services and had been convicted of firearms and drug offences. He shot his mother Maureen and later shot himself. His motives are unclear, but his long history of drug use may have contributed. Smoking skunk cannabis heavily was believed to have exacerbated Harris's schizophrenia. Prone to violent outbursts, he stabbed his long-term friend Carl James. Nandap stabbed Jeroen Ensink outside the victim's London house seemingly randomly. His sister had told police that high cannabis use was worsening his schizophrenia. At the time of the attack he was in a state of cannabis induced psychosis, perhaps falsely believing Ensink was a threat.

Motive and prevention

When a perpetrator has SMD, prevention can involve treating the apparent source of a motive through medication or other therapy. Falsely believed motivators may involve command hallucinations, conviction that the victim threatens the perpetrator, feelings of persecution and threat, a mission to kill, beliefs antipathetic to the victim, and broader animosity towards a wider group.

Where psychotic behaviour relates to drug use, preventive measures include the control of illegal drugs for the general population. It can also involve preventive strategies for the particular risk of self-administered drug abuse by people with SMD such as residential psychiatric care, and oversight in community settings.

With SCP approaches, motivation, which is sometimes side lined in the concentration on situational factors, can be relevant in some preventive scenarios. Situation and associated cues can influence the motive to carry out a specific type of crime. Consequently, where cues are removed and constraining preventive measures adopted, the level of motivation declines.

Within the framework of SCP, surveillance implies that perpetrators recognise degrees of risk. Even where someone acts on false beliefs or under a powerful obsession, surveillance can be preventive. It can range from treatment in a residential psychiatric setting to oversight in community facilities. These settings 'reduce anonymity' because those posing a risk are known to those treating them. They 'strengthen formal surveillance' and 'extend guardianship'. Less formally, approaches can 'assist natural surveillance'. Nandap's sister told police that his drug taking and watching conspiracy theory television shows was aggravating his mental disorder. However, the preventive power of her whistle blowing was not recognised.

'Reducing emotional arousal' can include controls of violent depictions on public media. Sometime before decapitating Anastasia Meshcheryakova, nanny Bobokulova had watched terrorist beheadings on the internet. 'Controlling drugs and alcohol' can be preventive where drug abuse has contributed to or triggered a psychotic episode.

Opportunity, homicide and SMD

Opportunity is a limited chance which involves a certain time or set of circumstances enabling something to be done. It is 'an occasion or situation that makes it possible to do something that you want to do or have to do' (Cambridge

University Press, 2020). An opportunity may arise either unsought or from a deliberate action.

Opportunity related to weapons

That opportunities for killing relates to the use of weapons was seen in the discussion on 'means' of killing. Weapons included ones that the perpetrator found at the scene and vehicles used intentionally to kill. Occasionally, means other than conventional weapons were used. Davydov fatally beat psychiatrist Wayne Fenton with his fists. Bobokulova manually strangled four-year-old Anastasia Meshcheryakova before beheading her. Diaz drowned her two young daughters in a bathtub at her home. Crook kicked, punched, and stamped on his elderly parents as well as hitting them with a hammer and strangling them with a belt.

Opportunity related to victims

Opportunity may arise for the perpetrator because the victims are vulnerable by age. Thaiday, Schloser, Diaz, and Laney killed their own children while Bobokulova killed a child in her care. Elderly parents were killed by Mark Tyler, and Timothy Crook. Lewis-Ranwell killed three elderly men who were strangers. Where victims are strangers to the perpetrator, the attack is likely to be unexpected, and the victim defenceless. This was so not only with Lewis-Ranwell, but with Nandap, Simelane, Devanov, Attias, and West.

Opportunity related undisturbed privacy

A private residence where the perpetrator is unlikely to be disturbed provides opportunity as with Lewis-Ranwell, Lacey, Bobokulova, Thaiday, Tyler, Crook, Bruce, Jones, Schloser, Diaz, Addy, and Dixon. Relatedly, Laney killed her young sons in the yard of her home in Texas. Also finding privacy, Carter killed Gino Nelmes in a halfway house run by a mental health support service. Davydov killed Wayne Fenton in the psychiatrist's private office, behind a locked door, alone, and at the weekend.

Opportunity related to sudden public attacks

When homicide occurs in a public place where others could intervene, opportunity typically arises from the suddenness and unexpectedness of the attack. Bonds shot officer Familia in her parked NYPD police vehicle at night and when she was occupied with paperwork. 'Out of the blue' Nandap stabbed Jeroen Ensink beside the victim's London house. Harris killed his life-long friend Carl James on the doorstep of the victim's home with a suddenness prohibiting any intervention. On a public bus, Simelane stabbed Christina Edkins and was able to disembark before other passengers realised what had happened. Devanov beheaded Jennifer Mills-Westley near a shop in Tenerife before anyone could step in. Driving his vehicle at speed into a group of young people, Attias killed four as they walked along a Santa Barbara roadside. West repeatedly ran her car over Jesus Plascencia in Los Angeles parking lot before anyone could prevent it.

Opportunity and prevention

Preventive strategies exist to minimise killings with certain weapons including controls on the sale of firearms, and police stop and search powers to reduce the incidence of carrying knives as offensive weapons. Where the victim is vulnerable by age, and the perpetrator is an employee, prevention may be possible. More thorough vetting of Nanny Bobokulova who killed a child in her care may have been possible.

Risks of privacy-related opportunity for homicide can be reduced where the venue for the killing is a workplace. Better supervision may have prevented Carter from killing Gino Nelmes in the house run by a mental health support service. Stronger security may have denied Davydov the opportunity to kill psychiatrist Wayne Fenton at the weekend, in the psychiatrist's private office, behind a locked door, and with no reliable third party being present. Another person being present might have stopped Dixon killing Ashleigh Ewing, visiting his home as an employee of a mental health charity.

Opportunity to commit a crime including homicide is a prominent feature of SCP which examines aspects of a situation increasing or reducing the opportunity to transgress. Being drivers of specific types of crime, altering or removing such situational encouragements can reduce opportunities to offend.

'Controlling tools or weapons' has already been discussed. 'Strengthening formal surveillance' includes improving the vetting of people employed to care for the vulnerable. Similarly, 'strengthening formal surveillance' is relevant in venues supervising people with SMD including community settings. It also applies to the self-protection of mental health workers such as Ashleigh Ewing, and psychiatrist Wayne Fenton.

Location of homicide

A location is a specified place or position. It can also refer to finding a place as when one speaks of 'locating' a person. A location can be a position or site identified by notable features or broad descriptions, or more precisely by co-ordinates.

Location and homicide in general

General homicide is patterned in space and time. A study analysed homicide location observed in three police forces in England and Wales 1994–1996 (Brookman, 2000). The commonest venue was a 'house' (52%), followed by 'street' (16%), 'open space' (15%), and 'public house/club' (9%). The 'house' could be that of the offender, or a friend – most common was the house of a victim or one shared by both offender and victim (Ibid.). Street, open space, and public house settings can involve a deadly mix of offensive exchanges, alcohol, public setting, and intense emotions or an argument. Home-based killings tend to involve intimate partner homicide, domestic violence, and the murder of loved ones or family (Richard Hough, 2017, personal communication).

Location, homicide and SMD

Crime location may be broadly described as a wide neighbourhood, or even more widely as an urban or rural setting. More precisely, location may be specified as a street, a building, or a room.

Residence shared by perpetrator and victim

Lisa Ann Diaz drowned her young daughters in a bathtub at their apartment in Plano, Texas. Dena Schloser amputated her baby daughter's arms also in a Plano apartment. Nathan Jones stabbed his mother Pamela with whom he lived at Mosby Woods, Sherman Street, City of Fairfax, USA. William Bruce killed his mother Amy as she worked at the desk in her home in Caratunk, Maine, USA.

At their shared home in Murray Street, Manoora, Cairns, Australia, Raina Mersane Ina Thaiday killed seven of her children and her niece. Mark Tyler shot his elderly mother Maureen at their shared home in Pitsea View Road, Cray's Hill, Basildon, Essex, England. Maureen Tyler's body was found on the living room sofa and Mark Tyler's in the en-suite bathroom. Marc Carter stabbed Gino Nelmes at their shared half-way house. A supported housing property in Filton Avenue, Bristol, England run by Keystones Mental Health Support Services, it was unsupervised at the weekend when the attack happened.

Timothy Crook killed his elderly parents in the home he shared with them in Swindon, Wiltshire, England. He then drove the bodies 150 miles away to Lincoln, depositing them in grounds of a house he owned. While her husband slept, Deana Laney killed her young sons at night in the yard of her home in New Chapel Hill, near Tyler, Texas.

Victim's residence (or occasionally workplace)

At night, Peter Atkins stabbed to death his son-in-law Stephen Provoost after breaking into his son-in-law and daughter's house in Rumney, Cardiff, Wales. Alexander Lewis-Ranwell killed Anthony Paine and twins Dick Carter and Roger Carter in their respective homes. Christian Lacey stabbed his mother Liz at her home in Hardy Street, Garston, Liverpool, England.

In the Moscow apartment of the child's parents, Gyulchekhra Boboku-lova killed Anastasia Meshcheryakova. Michael Harris stabbed his long-term friend Carl James on the doorstep of the victim's home in Swindon, Wiltshire, England. Gregory Davis killed Dorothy Rogers at her home on the Stantonbury Estate, Great Linford, Milton Keynes, England, then killed her son Michael after chasing him to a nearby playground. Patient Vitali Davydov beat to death psychiatrist Wayne Fenton in the doctor's office in Bethesda Maryland, USA.

Perpetrator's residence

Keith Michael Addy killed escort Annamarie Lewandowski in his apartment in 8700 block of W. National Avenue, West Allis, Milwaukee County, Wis-consin, USA. Ronald Dixon killed mental health worker Ashleigh Ewing when, alone, she visited his home in Heaton, Newcastle, England.

A public street or area

Percy Wright forcibly entered the home of former partner Colette Lynch and threatened her before chasing her from her home and fatally stabbing her out-side. Timchang Nandap stabbed Jeroen Ensink on the street outside the victim's London house. Near a shop in the resort of Los Christianos, Tenerife, Deyan Devanov ended the life of Jennifer Mills-Westley. David Attias drove his car at four young people on the 6500 block of Sabado Tarde Road in the Isla Vista neighbourhood near UCSB, Santa Barbara. Marie Elise West repeatedly ran her car over Jesus Plascencia in Van Nuys bagel shop parking lot, Los Angeles. After killing Dorothy Rogers at her home in Milton Keynes, Gregory Davis killed her son after chasing him to a nearby playground.

Inside a vehicle

Alexander Bonds shot police officer Familia in her NYPD vehicle parked at the corner of Morris Avenue and East 183rd Street New York City. As he disembarked an early morning public bus in Birmingham, England, Phillip Simelane stabbed schoolgirl Christina Edkins.

Location and prevention

Higher levels of supervision at the half-way house in which Marc Carter stabbed Gino Nelmes might have prevented the killing. The NYPD vehicle in which police officer Miosotis Familia was sitting when Alexander Bonds shot her might have been better protected for example by bullet proof windows. Had psychiatrist Wayne Fenton not seen patient Vitali Davydov alone in a small, locked private office, on a quiet weekend, he may not have been killed.

Ronald Dixon stabbed Ashleigh Ewing, an employee of a mental health charity, when she visited his home in Heaton, Newcastle, England without a third person, which might have prevented the attack. Better home security might have prevented Peter Atkins from killing his son-in-law Stephen Provoost after breaking into the victim's house in Rumney, Cardiff, Wales.

Concerning SCP and crime investigation, the location of a crime including homicide is often the starting point for evidence gathering and forensic work. In crime prevention, some locations may be identified as 'hot spots' for certain crimes. Strategies to reduce offending can involve analysing how a location might encourage it, then altering the location or aspects of it to reduce transgression.

Location can be used to protect a victim by 'hardening the target', for example through better supervision of property and physical protection. Examples are better supervision at the community setting where Gino Nelmes was killed; a third party being present with psychiatrist Wayne Fenton in his office; another person accompanying Ashleigh Ewing into Ronald Dixon's house; better home security for Stephen Provoost's home ('control access to facilities'); and bullet proof windows in officer Familia's NYPD vehicle.

It may have been preventive to 'avoid disputes' that contributed to Ashleigh Ewing being killed by Ronald Dixon, triggered by a debt letter she was delivering. A meeting might have been arranged at another site with several people present. Regarding 'reducing frustrations and stress', a locked and small private office perhaps adding to any stress and frustration felt by patient Vitali Davydov when he killed psychiatrist Wayne Fenton might have been avoided.

Interaction between means, motive, opportunity, and location

Means, motive, opportunity, and location can be interrelated, cumulatively aiding the perpetrating of a homicide. The examples of Dena Schloser and of Keith Michael Addy Illustrate this.

Dena Schloser

In January 2004, officials were called to the home of 39-year-old Dena Schloser in Plano, Dallas, Texas. She had been seen running down the street, with one of her daughters cycling after her. The child told officials that her mother had left her six-day-old sister alone in their apartment. Suffering from postpartum depression, Schloser appeared to be experiencing a psychotic episode and was hospitalized. She agreed to seek counselling and later saw a psychiatrist. Texas Child Protective Services carried out a seven-month investigation concluding that Schloser did not pose a risk to her children. Neighbours regarded her as a loving mother.

On 22 November 2004, Schloser was alone in the house with Margaret, her baby daughter. John Schlosser, her husband was at work and her two older daughters aged six and nine were attending school. That day, John Schloser telephoned a day-care centre and asked them to check on his wife and daughter.

Day-care workers telephoned his wife then called emergency services. When the 911 service called Dena Schloser, she told them that she had killed Margaret. On arriving at Schloser's apartment, police found the 11-month-old baby in her crib fatally injured while the mother was sitting in the living room covered in blood. Margaret was pronounced dead after arriving at hospital (Associated Press, 2004, 2015; Joyner, 2004; Religion News Blog, 2008).

Motive other than likely being related to a psychotic episode was unclear. However, the means of killing (a knife), the opportunity of being alone with a defenceless victim, and the location of the private apartment interrelated in allowing the homicide to take place. Had a weapon not been available, had the victim not been defenceless, had the apartment not been private, and had Schloser not been alone then the killing may have been averted.

Keith Michael Addy

Keith Michael Addy, 26, was a former sex offender. Reports are unclear about his social background and employment status. On Thursday 6 March 2003 Addy rang an agency 'Beautiful Blondes' and asked for an escort to come to his apartment in West Allis, Milwaukee County, Wisconsin where he was alone. Annamarie Lewandowski, 19 and the mother of a one-year-old baby duly arrived. Addy put a hood over her head, tied her up, and dripped hot wax on her.

Then he repeatedly hit her over the head with a framing hammer, and finally repeatedly stabbed her. An hour later, using a saw, he dismembered her body in the bathtub. Putting the body parts in bags, Addy disposed of them in trash, with the help of an unwitting neighbour. Before leaving for the job, Lewandowski had left the details and address with Jacqueline Lewandowski her roommate (and cousin) who called the police the next day when Ann Marie had failed to return.

Police searched Addy's premises and discovered the body parts in the trash. Addy told detectives that voices ordered him to kill Lewandowski and that he was possessed by demons. It was reported that Addy experienced an unrecognised mental disorder for a year before the killing (Fox6News, 2018; Milwaukee County Case 2003CF001468; Vielmetti, 2018).

Addy's motive which he claimed was not sexual, was likely sadistic. The means of bludgeoning with a hammer and stabbing with a knife, the opportunity of being alone with the escort, and the location of his apartment allowing him to be undisturbed again combined to enable the killing.

Conclusions

Means of homicide by perpetrators with SMD may involve using edge weapons, beating, and bludgeoning, strangulation, the use of firearms, driving a vehicle, drowning, and using multiple means. Perpetrators may use available in situ weapons or ones taken to the scene, and the killing may implicate excessive and dramatic violence. Motives may involve command hallucinations, animosity towards the victim or wider group, conviction that the victim threatens the perpetrator, beliefs antipathetic to the victim, general feelings of persecution and threat, a mission to kill, and unclear possibly drug related motives. Opportunity may relate to weapons, the victim, undisturbed privacy, and sudden public attack. Location may be the residence shared by perpetrator and victim, the victim's home or workplace, the perpetrator's residence, a public street/area, and inside a vehicle.

With many preventive techniques there are limitations such as the expense involved in protecting pedestrians from the rare instances of intentional vehicle injury. Authorities must weigh the odds of potential crimes and use whatever preventive steps are practicable. There are rarely easy solutions. Preventive techniques emerging from SCP and relevant to means, motive, opportunity, and location are as follows.

- Using roadside barriers in selected high-risk busy city areas to protect pedestrians from deliberate vehicle attacks.
- Limiting access to firearms through purchaser background checks, seizing illegally imported firearms, and confiscating offensive edge weapons through police 'stop and search' powers.
- Providing timely psychiatric treatment including, where appropriate, therapy addressing motivational false beliefs.
- Stopping access to internet violent depictions.
- Controlling access to drugs and alcohol contributing to violence or psychotic episodes.
- Improved vetting of people working with vulnerable individuals
- Better supervision and care of residents with SMD in community settings.
- Highlighting better self-protection for mental health workers seeing high risk patients such as having a third-party present and avoiding enclosed spaces.
- Effective safety procedures if workers visit the homes of people with SMD.
- Stronger police vehicle protection such as bullet proof windows

Suggested activities

Select from the glossary a case and consider the means, motive, opportunity, and location involved. To what extent do they relate to each other? For example, is the opportunity for homicide aided by the location? Does the motive for the killing influence the means chosen? Select a second case and carry out the same analysis. Compare and contrast the findings to develop your understanding of the possible relationships between these features.

Read the report in the 'Key texts' section concerning Ronald Dixon's killing of Ashleigh Ewing. Consider how means, motive, opportunity, and location influenced the homicide.

Key texts

NHS England (2013) *Report to NHS England of the Independent Investigation into the Healthcare and Treatment of 'Patient P'* (Commissioned by the Former North East Strategic Health Authority) http://hundredfamilies.org/wp/wp-content/uploads/2013/12/ RONALD_DIXON_May06.pdf.

This report relates to the killing of Ashleigh Ewing, an employee of a mental health charity by Ronald Dixon. It can be read with a focus on how the means, opportunity, and location (and possible the motive) relates to a homicide.

References

Associated Press (23 November 2004 and 4 January 2015) 'Cops: Mother cut off baby's arms' *Fox News* www.foxnews.com/story/cops-mother-cut-off-babys-arms.

Australian Associated Press (2017) 'Mother psychotic when she killed eight children, Queensland court rules' *Guardian* (4 May 2017) www.theguardian.com/australia-news/2017/may/04/mother-psychotic-when-she-killed-eight-children-queensland-court-rules.

Barr, C. W., Londoño, E. and Morse, D. (2006) 'Patient admits killing psychiatrist, police say' *Washington Post* (5 September 2006) www.washingtonpost.com/wp-dyn/content/ article/2006/09/04/AR2006090400430.html.

BBC News (2003) 'Mother and son killed by "psychotic"' BBC News (15 December 2003) http://news.bbc.co.uk/1/hi/england/beds/bucks/herts/3322525.stm.

BBC News (2013) 'Mental health review after Cray's Hill double death incident' BBC News (27 March 2013) www.bbc.co.uk/news/uk-england-essex-21951670.

BBC News (2015) 'Manslaughter: Timothy Crook guilty of killing parents' BBC News (20 July 2015) www.bbc.co.uk/news/uk-england-wiltshire-33599525.

Bernstein, E. and Koppel, N. (2008) 'A death in the family' *Wall Street Journal* (16 August 2008) www.wsj.com/articles/SB121883750650245525.

Brookman, F. (2000) *Dying for Control: Men, Murder and Sub-Lethal Violence in England and Wales.* Unpublished PhD Thesis, Cardiff University.

Cambridge University Press (2020) *Cambridge Dictionary.* https://dictionary.cambridge.org/ dictionary/english/opportunity.

Celona, L. and Golding, B. (2017) 'NYPD cop-killer was a schizophrenic off his meds: Girlfriend' *New York Post* (5 July 2017) https://nypost.com/2017/07/05/nypd-cop-killer-was-a-schizophrenic-off-his-meds-girlfriend/.

Clarke, R. V. (2018) 'The Theory and Practice of Situational Crime Prevention' Criminology and Criminal Justice Oxford Research Encyclopaedias On-line publication (January 2018) https://oxfordre.com/criminology/view/10.1093/acrefore/9780190264079.001.0001/acrefore-9780190264079-e-327#acrefore-9780190264079-e-327-div2-3.

Docking, N. (21 December 2018) 'Man stabbed his mum to death and tried to kill his gran's carer in psychotic episode' *Echo* (21 December 2018) www.liverpoolecho.co.uk/ news/liverpool-news/christian-lacey-liz-lacey-murder-15584632.

Ellis, T. M. and Emily, J. (2006) 'Child-killer to leave hospital' *The Dallas Morning News* (10 November 2006) www.pressreader.com/usa/the-dallas-morning-news/20061110/281552286359490.

Evans, M. (2018) 'Widow of academic stabbed to death on his doorstep demands to know why psychotic knifeman was released to kill' *Telegraph* (2 July 2018) www.telegraph. co.uk/news/2018/07/02/psychotic-killer-attacked-new-father-told-police-leave-dead/.

Falkenberg, L. (2003) 'Closing arguments begin in Texas mother's murder trial' *Associated Press* (3 April 2003) www.cephas-library.com/assembly_of_god/ assembly_of_ god_member_killed _her_sons.html.

Farrell, M. (2017) *Criminology of Homicidal Poisoning: Offenders, Victims and Detection*. London and New York, Springer.

Federal Bureau of Investigation (2018) United States 2018 Uniform Crime Reports Homicide Data 'Expanded Homicide Data Table 7 Murder Types of Weapons Used 2018' Washington DC, Federal Bureau of Investigation. https://ucr.fbi.gov/crime-in-the-u.s/2018/crime-in-the-u.s.-2018/tables/expanded-homicide-data-table-7.xls.

Fox6News (2018) 'Man who killed teen, dismembered her body could be released from mental health facility soon'. www.dailymotion.com/video/x6hmen7.

Gilligan, A. (2013) 'Truth about dangerous mental patients let out to kill' *The Telegraph* (5 October 2013) www.telegraph.co.uk/news/uknews/crime/10358251/Truth-about-dangerous-mental-patients-let-out-to-kill.html.

Joyner, J. (2004) 'Mom cut off baby's arms' *Outside the Beltway* (23 November 2004) www.outsidethebeltway.com/mom_cut_off_babys_arms/.

Lagos, M. (2002) 'Jury finds Attias guilty of murder' *Daily Nexus* (6 June 2002) http:// dailynexus.com/2002-06-06/jury-finds-attias-guilty-of-murder/.

Matejkowski, J. C., Cullen, S. W. and Solomon, P. L. (2008) 'Characteristics of persons with severe mental illness who have been incarcerated for murder' *Journal of the American Academy of Psychiatry and the Law*, 36, 74–86.

Milwaukee County Case 2003CF001468 *State of Wisconsin vs. Keith Michael Addy*. https://wcca.wicourts.gov/caseDetail.html?cacheId=19D57A47CFCA121AB4538508 BF3315A7&caseNo=2003CF001468&countyNo=40&mode=details&offset=11& recordCount=12#summary.

Minero, V. A., Barker, E. and Bedford, R. (2017) 'Method of homicide and severe mental illness: a systematic review' *Aggression and Violent Behavior*, 37, 52–62.

Morris, S. (2019) 'Killer of three elderly Devon men found not guilty of murder due to insanity' *The Guardian* (2 December 2019) www.theguardian.com/uk-news/2019/ dec/02/killer-of-three-elderly-devon-men-found-not-guilty-due-to-insanity.

NHS England (2013) *Report to NHS England of the Independent Investigation into the Healthcare and Treatment of 'Patient P'* (Commissioned by the Former North East Strategic Health Authority) http://hundredfamilies.org/wp/wp-content/uploads/ 2013/12/ RONALD_DIXON_May06.pdf.

Parker, B. L. and McKinley, A. C. (2018) 'Homicide event motive: A situational perspective' *Salus Journal* 6, 2, 78–95.

Pelletier, K. (2017) *Motivation to Kill: The Relationship between Motive and Weapon Choice in Homicide* (Masters dissertation, Arizona State University) https://repository. asu.edu/ attachments/ 186614/content/Pelletier_asu_0010N_16832.pdf.

Petri, H. L. and Cofer, C. N. (2019) 'Motivation' *Encyclopaedia Britannica* (6 June 2019).

Policeone.com (accessed 2020) www.policeone.com/edged-weapons/.

Religion News Blog (2008) 'Dean Schlosser who cut off baby's arms moving to outpatient care' *Religion News Blog* (12 November 2008) www.religionnewsblog.com/ 22921/dena-schlosser.

Reporter (3 April 2006) 'Paranoid schizophrenic Marc Carter jailed for Bristol Samurai sword killing of Gino Nelmes' *HuffPost* (1 February 2013) and updated (3 April 2013) www.huffingtonpost.co.uk/2013/02/01/pranoid-schizophrenic-man2599343.html.

Reporter (2 August 2007) 'Schizophrenic addicted to skunk cannabis killed best friend' *Evening Standard* (2 August 2007) www.standard.co.uk/news/schizophrenic-addicted-to-skunk-cannabis-killed-best-friend-6602755.html.

Reporter (18 December 2007) 'Jones found not guilty by reason of insanity' *The Connection* (18 December 2007) www.connectionnewspapers.com/ news/2007/dec/18/jones-not-guilty-by-reason-of-insanity/.

Savill, R. (2001) 'Son-in-law stabbed to death in marital bed' *The Telegraph* (6 June 2001) www.telegraph.co.uk/news/uknews/1311615/Son-in-law-stabbed-to-death-in-marital-bed.html.

Shaw, J., Amos, T., Hunt, I. M. and Flynn, S, Turnbull, P., Kapur, N. and Appleby, L. (2004) 'Mental illness in people who kill strangers: Longitudinal study and national clinical survey' *BMJ*, 328:734–737.

TASS (2016) 'The murder of a child in Moscow: Investigation progress and public reaction' TASS (29 February 2016) https://tass.ru/proisshestviya/2706157 (in Russian).

Teetor, P. (2002) 'Prelude to a death' *Los Angeles Times* (5 May 2002) www.latimes.com/archives/la-xpm-2002-may-05-tm-41435-story.html.

Twomey, J. (2009) 'Fury after psychotic killer walks free after four years' *Express* (22 April 2002) www.express.co.uk/news/uk/96406/Fury-as-psychotic-killer-walks-free-after-4-years.

Vielmetti, B. (2018) 'Man who killed, dismembered woman denied release from mental hospital' *Milwaukee Journal Sentinel* (16 April 2018) https://eu.jsonline.com/story/news/crime/2018/04/12/man-who-killed-dismembered-woman-2003-denied-release-mental-hospital/511533002/.

Welton, B. (2013) 'Birmingham bus killer Philip Simelane to be held at a psychiatric unit indefinitely' *Manchester Evening News* (2 October 2013) www.manchestereveningnews.co.uk/news/uk-news/birmingham-bus-killer-phillip-simelane-6128265.

Chapter 8

Organisational constraints on prevention

Introduction

When considering how a homicide perpetrated by an individual with SMD might have been prevented (or the risk of it mitigated) the organisation of services and issues such as their communication systems can be important. After such incidents, inquiries may be carried out and reports produced. Philip Simelane's killing of Christina Edkins led to reports in 2014 and in 2017. Marc Carter's stabbing of Gino Nelmes was followed by a report of 2014. But what do such documents and the inquiries behind them contribute to understanding whether the risk of homicide could have been reduced? How relevant are they to reducing the risks of future homicides?

Other cases also illustrate organisational and communication problems including in multi-agency working between the many groups involved such as police, mental health services, social services, courts, and prisons. There can be insufficient clarity about the roles and responsibilities of staff in various agencies and services. So-called longitudinal views of a perpetrator's background can be given too little attention. Not enough credence may be given to the concerns of the perpetrator's family and carers. It may not be recognised that effective psychiatric treatment including sufficient psychiatric beds is necessary. It is these issues with which this chapter is mainly concerned. But first it touches on examples where organisational issues were not central.

Organisations and services that can have contact with people with SMD

Numerous organisations and services can have (sometimes prolonged) contact with individuals with SMD. Among these are health services (physicians, nurses), mental health services (psychiatrists, psychiatric nurses), community psychiatric teams, staff working in 'half-way houses' and other community based facilities for people with mental disorders, prison services (prison officers, rehabilitation staff), probation services, court personnel, police (arresting officers, custody officers), mental health charities, staff supporting the homeless including

DOI: 10.4324/9781003172727-10

in homeless shelters, social workers, and many others. Their work can be under great time pressure and in highly stressful situations.

Cases not centring on organisational failure

Cases where there were few or no indications of SMD prior to the homicide

Prior to her killings, Riana Thaiday had never been treated for mental illness. Neighbours seemingly noticed Thaiday's strange behaviour ten days before the killings. Several psychiatrists testified after the event that her mental state likely deteriorated in the months before the deaths (Australian Associated Press, 2017).

A year before bludgeoning to death her children Deana Laney told fellow church members that the world was ending, and that God had ordered her to get her house in order. After the killings, Laney claimed that God told her to do it. Neighbours viewed the family as stable and loving and Laney had no documented history of mental disorder (Falkenberg, 2003).

Keith Michael Addy bludgeoned, stabbed, and dismembered an escort that he had paid through an agency to visit his house. A former sex offender, it is reported that Addy experienced an unrecognised mental disorder for a year before the killing. He told detectives that voices commanded him to kill Lewandowski and that he was possessed by demons (Milwaukee County Case 2003CF001468).

David Attias deliberately ran over and killed four pedestrians with his car. Before the killing he is reported to have had mental health and drug problems. After running over the victims, Attias climbed on top of his vehicle and declared that he was, 'the angel of death'. Blood tests indicated that he was under the influence of marijuana and Lidocaine, but these were not deemed influential in the incident. There were seemingly no clear indications of the impending violence (Lagos, 2002).

Cases where services had been involved but homicide probably could not be foreseen

Around 4am on 12 May 2006 Mrs Jones called her estranged husband saying that their son Nathan was acting psychotically and refusing his medication. About 7 am Mr Jones looked in and drove Nathan to a nearby park, telling him to take his medication on returning home. Later Nathan, away from home and speaking incoherently, contacted his father who became concerned and picked him up to go home. Entering the house Mr Jones found his wife's body where Nathan had stabbed her. Prevention was hindered because Nathan's parents were not mental health professionals and events rapidly got worse (Reporter, 18 December 2007).

In January 2004, authorities were called to Dena Schloser's home. Appearing to be suffering postpartum depression and having a psychotic episode, she was hospitalized. Texas Child Protective Services held a seven-month investigation concluding Schloser pose no risk to her children. Neighbours regarded her as a loving mother and there was no family history of violence. In November 2004, Schloser killed her baby daughter Margaret (Joyner, 2004).

Gregory Davis stabbed a female acquaintance and her son. In 2003, after the killing, he was diagnosed with depression, alcohol dependence, and social anxiety. In his diary, he had recorded plans to become a serial killer, but everyone seemed ignorant of these aspirations (BBC News, 2003).

Peter Atkins had schizophrenia for many years. He suspected his wife of having an affair and developed animosity towards his son-in-law. In July 2000, he argued with his daughter and her husband, and cut the petrol pipe on her car. On 24 January 2001, Atkin's wife Carol called police to their home after Atkins had punched and kicked her because the kitchen was messy. Next day, Atkins killed his son-in-law, afterwards telling police, 'It did not seem real to me. It was like a dream' (Savill, 2001).

Marie Elise West deliberately and repeatedly ran over a man in her car in January 2001. Years before, she had enrolled in law school but left owing to mental health problems. Diagnosed with bipolar disorder in 1990, in the following ten years West was arrested six times and hospitalised 19 times. On the evening of the killing, she resisted her husband's efforts to persuade her to check in at the facility at Harbor-UCLA and went to her job waitressing. After acting erratically, West was sent home from work, where she began obsessing that a certain Michael Maglieri, the son of a club owner, would be killed by gang members. At 11.30 pm she left in her car saying she was going to rescue Maglieri. Despite her long-standing mental disorder, it is difficult to see how the killing could have been foreseen (Teetor, 2002).

In these instances, organisational problems do not appear central. At one end of the spectrum, SMD may have been the first episode to occur so that relatives, neighbours, and others were unaware. Authorities may not have been informed. At the opposite end of the intervention pole, authorities may have been involved for years and the incidents around the time of the killing may have been no different to ones that had not led to extreme violence in the past.

In some other cases, as will now be explored, organisational issues are more central.

Phillip Simelane's killing of Christina Edkins

Events around the death

On 7 March 2013 around 5.00 am, Philip Simelane boarded a bus near the city centre in Birmingham, England and went to the upper deck where he fell asleep. Christina Edkins got on the bus around 7.30 am and also sat on the upper deck. Almost immediately, Simelane rose and moved forward three seats and sat down again. Removing a knife from his bag, he hid it against his leg. He then rose and walked towards Edkins' seat, stabbed her and disembarked. Emergency services attended but Edkins was pronounced dead at around 8 am. Simelane was arrested a few hours later and told police that he had bought the knife the previous day, fearing for his own safety. Simelane and Edkins were strangers. Convicted of manslaughter on the grounds of diminished responsibility, Simelane was detained in a secure psychiatric hospital.

Phillip Simelane had previously been in prison. His mental health problems began in his mid-teens when he had several criminal convictions including two knife offences. At trial, the judge expressed concern that Simelane was not receiving treatment at the time of the killing (Welton, 2013).

Reports following the death

In September 2014, the Birmingham and Solihull Mental Health NHS Foundation Trust published a report following an investigation into the circumstances of Christina Edkins' death. The report (Reed, 2014) identified 'Overarching lessons learned' (Ibid., section 6.2). These included that some of the services and departments involved in Simelane's care did not hold a review of their involvement 'to identify lessons learned'. When services are designed and put into practice, it should be recognised that people with mental disorder may not have the mental capacity to initiate or take part in their care. Organisations providing services failed to adequately 'listen to, respond to, and support' carers and others. Arrangements for recording and storing information were not robust enough to assist good care and management. Key agencies were ineffective in accessing and sharing information; for example, the general practitioner was not 'consistently updated'. Longitudinal perspectives on assessment and management were not fully used in 'sound decision making and the provision of care' (Ibid., partly paraphrased).

Among 'Significant points and lessons learned' was an issue relating to courts and sentencing. In an earlier offence when Simelane jabbed a knife at his mother's stomach in the presence of his younger brother and was arrested for threats to kill. However, the Police National Computer records showed sentencing for an offence of battery, resulting in a short custody of 26 weeks, and limiting the time available to arrange for Simelane's possible admission to hospital. The report highlights a different inquiry (of 1994) stating that when charging a person with 'mental illness' the charge should reflect the seriousness of the offence (Reed, 2014, section 6.9 para 1, pp. 80–81).

Recommendations were also made for organisations (Ibid., summary table 4). These concerned the NHS foundation Trust, the Mental Health NHS Foundation Trust, the Her Majesty's Prison and related Health and Care NHS Trusts, General Practitioners, Police, and Social Services (Ibid., pp. 84–88). Other national level recommendations were made for organisations and services including the Crown Prosecution Service, courts, the Ministry of Justice, and the Department of Health (Ibid., p. 89).

For example, staff working in prison with responsibility for 'assessment or management of cases' should plan for prisoner discharges 'from an early stage' and liaise with relevant providers and agencies having 'responsibility for the final assessment prior to release' (p. 87 point 4, partly paraphrased).

A second report into the care and treatment of Simelane in the West Midlands was issued in 2017 (Jenkins and Moor, 2017). Its forward states,

> The absence of access to partner organisations' IT systems, information sharing, joined up thinking and working practice as well as longitudinal assessment, all contributed to the failings identified in this case. ... They have been identified as the root cause of failures in the past and continue to be identified as root causes of failures today.
>
> (Ibid., p. 4)

Recommendations were made considering what had already been implemented following the earlier report. These included 'priority 1' recommendations which were considered fundamental. For example, one relating to Her Majesty's Prison Hewell (Healthcare) and HMP Birmingham (Healthcare) was that,

> Staff undertaking the initial Care Programme Approach Plan must ensure that they liaise with all agencies who have been involved with the prisoner, in the community and/or during the court process ... to obtain an accurate profile of their needs and risks to themselves and others.
>
> (Jenkins and Moor, 2017, p. 24)

Prevention and reducing risk of homicide

Predictability is rarely going to be possible as, if it were, attacks would be stopped. In making risk assessments, psychiatrists and others do not try to predict that a homicide will take place, because this is not possible. They set out the risks and the increased risks of such an event. The key question then is preventability. Events can of course be prevented even when they are not predicted.

In the 2014 report into the death of Christina Edkins (Reed, 2014, section 5, pp. 72–73) the investigation panel concluded that there were several opportunities, 'where mental health treatment and follow-up could have been established'. They noted that Simelane's, 'history of violence to others had been escalating and he had been known to be in possession of knives and made reference in public to stabbing'. The panel maintained that the homicide was 'directly related' to Simelane's mental illness and 'could have been prevented if his mental health needs had been identified and met'.

Marc Carter's killing of Gino Nelmes

Events around the death

On 17 March 2012 Marc Carter fatally stabbed Gino Nelmes with a samurai sword in a Keystones shared house, Bristol. Keystones is a Mental Health Support Service. Nelmes had lived in the house for some years.

For the previous year, Carter had been a patient at Fromeside Medium Secure Unit, Bristol and was on trial leave at the Keystones house. He had previously been admitted to high and medium secure hospitals and imprisoned for serious assaults. He had a diagnosis of 'paranoid schizophrenia' (schizophrenia with delusions of persecution). In September 2011 it was reported that Carter 'had 29 convictions relating to 61 crimes' including 'offences against people and property'. He was said to use drugs including 'cannabis, amphetamines, heroin, crack cocaine, LSD, magic mushrooms and solvents' (Niche, 2014, section 7.4.5).

Carter had moved into Keystones on 5 March 2012 following two short trial periods. During an earlier stay it is believed that Carter had smoked cannabis and, on a trip to Newport, had acquired the Samurai sword used to attack Nelmes. As a result of Carter using cannabis on an earlier stay, the Fromeside multidisciplinary team delayed his discharge and decided to continue trial leave with increased supervision from mental health staff.

On Saturday 17 March 2012 both Carter and Nelmes were in the facility. The Keystones director arrived shortly before 4pm for a meeting in the office at the top of the house and met her visitor at the front door five minutes later. Carter later told psychiatrists that he felt that Nelmes could read his thoughts and was laughing at him. Carter went to his bedroom (next to the kitchen on the ground floor) got his sword and stabbed Nelmes. The exact time is unknown. At 5.10pm an on-call staff member told the director that she had received a telephone call from a resident saying that Nelmes was injured. An ambulance was called but Nelmes died on arrival at hospital. Carter was missing but shortly afterwards reported to a police station. He later pleaded guilty to manslaughter on the grounds of diminished responsibility and was sentenced to a minimum of 12 years imprisonment; he was transferred to a psychiatric hospital. The facility was fully supervised during the week but not at the weekend when the attack took place (Reporter, 3 April 2006; Niche, 2014).

Report on the homicide

A report into the events was published in 2014 (Niche, 2014). The purpose of the investigation was to, 'Identify whether there were any aspects of the care which could have altered or prevented the incident. The investigation process will also identify areas where improvements to services might be required which could help prevent similar incidents occurring' (Niche, 2014, section 3, p. 9).

The report (Niche, 2014) referred to an earlier investigation conducted by Avon and Wiltshire Mental Health Partnership NHS Trust which noted that risk assessment documentation was incomplete; and a community care plan (including a crisis and contingency plan) was not detailed enough. Also, the electronic patient record risk assessment and core assessment did not adequately reflect that Carter had been convicted of a 'Multi-Agency Public Protection Arrangements' (MAPPA) eligible offence. (In England and Wales, such protection arrangements concern authorities, for example police, probation, and prison services, involved in managing certain offenders, including ones posing a serious risk of harm to the public). In Carter's case, a relevant group were not informed when he started leave and his discharge was planned (Ibid., p. 5 point 3, partly paraphrased).

The Niche report of 2014 included recommendations around multi-disciplinary working, sharing information, planning, and the use of risk assessments. For example, the Trust should, 'ensure that, in forensic services, there is a multi-disciplinary discussion and agreement on individual, evidence-based risk assessment, including static, dynamic and personality factors, and a clear link between risk assessment and risk management' (Niche, 2014, p. 58, item 3).

The report argued that Carter should have passed through the various wards (with different levels of security) at Fromeside more slowly. This would have enabled more rigorous testing of 'risk indicators and his management of these' and 'his use of illicit substances, in particular cannabis and its effects on his mental state' (Niche, 2014, p. 32, section 9.1.2).

At weekends when the attack took place staff supervision was light. A staff member would call into each house briefly twice a day and speak to all those in the house. There is someone on call 24 hours a day and an evening security visit (Niche, 2014, p. 17 paraphrased).

The report does not appear to have uncovered how Carter got the Samurai sword (it was possibly on a trip to Newport), who knew that he had it, and why it was considered safe to keep it on the property.

Organisational and related preventive strategies: cases from 2000 to 2020

Implications of **indications of accumulating risk including** the period shortly before **Lewis-Ranwell** killed seem to have been missed. Potential red flags were his committing burglary, his threatening a farmer, his mother's worried telephone call to police about her son's release, and police concerns about the risk to the public. **No overarching assessment** brought these indications together. At his trial, the jury raised concerns with the judge about the 'state of psychiatric services' in Devon and the 'failings in care'. Devon Partnership and Devon County Council both involved in the case said they would learn lessons (Morris, 2019).

Missed opportunities in 2018 were the 30 March **misreading** of **Christian Lacey's symptoms** at the Royal Liverpool Hospital, and the assessment by Merseycare staff that he did not need to be 'sectioned' into psychiatric care. A review of the case found that staff **failed to enquire** why Lacey had attacked his father and half-brother. Some Criminal Justice Liaison Team members had not received formal training in mental health before joining the team. Practitioners did not explore Lacey's complex presentation in enough depth. Subsequently, Merseycare ordered new training in recognising psychosis and in assessing risks, and reminders to employees to properly question the family and carers of mental health patients (Docking, 2018).

When **Alexander Bonds** killed a police officer in her vehicle, **better physical safety precautions** such as bullet proof windows could have been preventive (Celona and Golding, 2017).

Nanny **Gyulchekhra Bobokulova** had been treated for schizophrenia years before she killed, but any reservations about her working with vulnerable people were not **shared with other agencies.** Relatedly, systems to recruit, register, monitor, and supervise workers with vulnerable people were insufficient (TASS, 2016).

Earlier identification of the **accumulating potential risk** around **Timchang Nandap** may have led to his being treated in psychiatric provision. Risk indicators included Nandap's arrest in May 2015 wielding a knife on a London street where his sister lived, his **sister's call to police** saying that Nandap's high cannabis use and watching conspiracy theories on television were worsening his condition, and her warning that he was experiencing 'paranoia' and hallucinations and should not be interviewed alone; **arresting officers noticing** Nandap behaving strangely possibly owing to drug abuse or mental illness; a doctor examining Nandap before the interview claiming that he was **given no 'markers'** on his mental health; seeming missed information on the custody record; Nandap answering strangely when interviewed; **no Merlin report** being created on Nandap, so mental health concerns not highlighted to others; and Nandap's clinical treatment in Nigeria for psychosis including hallucinations (Evans, 2018).

As was seen earlier in the chapter, regarding **Phillip Simelane**, organisations providing services did not adequately **listen to, respond to, and support carers** and others. Key agencies were **ineffective in accessing and sharing information**. Lack of access to partner organisations computer systems, information sharing, and working practice, contributed to failings. Prison staff and others concerned with Simelane's discharge **did not liaise fully** enough to prepare for his release. Longitudinal perspectives on **assessment and management were not fully used** to aid sound decision making and care provision. Simelane's **escalating violence** including threats of stabbing were insufficiently recognised. His mental health needs were not identified and met (Reed, 2014).

Mark Tyler shot his mother, then days later himself. In 2010 he was convicted of firearms and drug offences and had a long history of drug abuse. Between February 2011 and July 2012 Tyler had four mental health assessments but was not diagnosed with a specific condition. In July 2012, he attended a health assessment/psychiatric consultation, but seemingly no diagnosis was made. A domestic homicide review into the case by Basildon Community Safety published in November 2015 found that Tyler exhibited bizarre behaviour. His mother resisted attempts by family members to take Tyler to hospital, believing that she could care for him. The report recommended **better sharing of information and a more multi-agency approach** to provide comprehensive support (BBC, 2013).

On 17 March 2012 in a mental health 'half-way house', **Marc Carter** on 'leave' arrangements from Fromeside, a medium secure facility, fatally stabbed Gino Nelmes. Subsequent inquiries indicated weaknesses in **multidisciplinary working and information sharing**. This contributed to a relevant group not being informed when Carter started his 'leave' and his discharge was planned. Carter may have passed too quickly through Fromeside's various wards with different levels of security, limiting opportunity to better test **risk indicators** and how Carter dealt with them.

A 'drifter' who killed a stranger in Tenerife, **Deyan Devanov** had been 'sectioned' at his family's request as an involuntary inpatient at a mental health unit in North Wales. He was released in October 2010. A Health Inspectorate of Wales enquiry report of November 2014 found that Devanov was **misdiagnosed as faking mental illness** before his release from the unit. Devanov may have acted on command hallucinations of heard voices telling him to kill. He was said to take cocaine and LSD (Gilligan, 2013).

Michael Harris who killed his life-long friend, had schizophrenia and was prone to violent outbursts. He heavily smoked skunk cannabis, exacerbating his schizophrenia. At the trial defence lawyers stated that mental health workers had been aware of Harris's problems but did not intervene. A report commissioned by the Strategic Health Authority criticised the Avon and Wiltshire Partnership NHS Trust for the poor treatment and lack of management direction which contributed to the death of the victim. It stated that there was **'an accumulation of poor practice'** and **'failures in systems'** and a **lack of 'managerial direction and control'**. These were causal factors in the victim's death (Reporter, 2 August 2007).

'Sectioned' in 2002, **Timothy Crook** had been diagnosed with 'paranoid schizophrenia' (now 'schizophrenia with delusions of persecution'). After being discharged, he refused contact with mental health services and declined to take his medication. At some point Crook believed that police were conspiring against him and that he was being pursued by US forces. However, the exact motive for the killing of his parents is unclear. Preventative strategies could have included **better recognition of the risk** of Crook's **not taking medication and contact with mental health services and developing approaches to better ensure this**. Crook's sister Janice Lawrence claims that she contacted Avon and Wiltshire Mental Health Trust prior to the killing to alert them to **concerns about her brother** (BBC News, 2015).

Psychiatrist Wayne Fenton was killed by **Vitali Davydov** who was not his regular patient, had schizophrenia, and was declining to take his anti-psychotic medication. Dr Fenton saw the patient in a small office seemingly behind a locked door. The patient's father had left to run an errand and Dr Fenton was alone with the patient and it was a weekend, a quieter time than weekdays. Risk of violence to the clinician increases when severely ill, psychotic patients are seen alone, especially at evenings or on weekends. Clinicians should have a reliable third party present for the initial evaluation of an unknown patient with SMD. **Better physical and procedural safety precautions** may have been preventive (Barr, Londoño, and Morse, 2006).

Having a history of mental disorder, **Ronald Dixon** had been detained in psychiatric care, diagnosed with symptoms of schizophrenia and mania. A December 2005 review by a consultant and a community psychiatric nurse missed the opportunity to increase monitoring of Dixon and clarify inter-agency roles. A month later, he was arrested outside Buckingham Palace saying he would kill the Queen. He was returned to Newcastle and held in a secure unit but not assessed while displaying psychotic symptoms. Following a risk assessment in February 2006 he was discharged to supported accommodation. By May there had been 'significant changes' in Dixon's presentation but no community psychiatric nurse formally reviewed his care. There had been a **lack of overarching assessment** and indications of **accumulating risk** were missed. On 19 May 2006, Dixon killed a lone, female employee of a mental health charity who was visiting his home. Questions were raised about the **adequacy of safety procedures** (NHS England, 2013).

William Bruce was diagnosed with paranoid schizophrenia in 2005 after a series of violent incidents. These included that, while in a hunting party, he turned a gun on his father and two friends (although he did not shoot them). After this incident he was admitted to Acadia Hospital, Bangor, Maine. Following another attack on his father on 6 February 2006, Bruce was placed in Riverview Psychiatric Recovery Center, Maine from where he was discharged on 20 April 2006. Two months later, he killed his mother. **Bruce's father believed that his son should not have been released** from Riverview Psychiatric Recovery Center in April 2006 and blamed patient advocates for pressing for Bruce's release (Bernstein and Koppel, 2008).

Services including police did not respond rigorously enough to **signs of increased risk** in the case of **Percy Wright**. By January 2005, his mental health was getting worse and Colette Lynch, his former partner, warned his doctor of his becoming 'paranoid and aggressive'. Wright told his general practitioner that he was hearing voices. On 1 February 2005, Wright forced his way into Lynch's home, attacking her and threatening to cut her throat, but she escaped. At 11.30pm that night a nurse twice telephoned police. She informed police Wright had left hospital (after treatment for injuries sustained breaking into Lynch's house), that his mental health was getting worse, and that she considered him a threat to Lynch. Police failed to arrest Wright or record the incident as a crime and failed to follow their domestic violence policy. Next night Wright was assessed by a social worker outside his house and judged fit to remain there. Before a planned formal assessment could be carried out Wright killed his victim (Twomey, 2009).

Lisa Ann Diaz drowned her two young daughters. Opportunities seem to have been missed to **recognise accumulating risk indicators and declining mental health**. From 2002, Diaz reported experiencing many ailments, making numerous visits to doctors or alternative therapists. She developed an increasing obsessive fear of germs, believing that she had transmitted her illnesses to her children. On 2 September 2003, Diaz saw a physician who suggested her problems were psychosomatic and referred her to a Dallas psychiatrist whom subsequently she did not see. At the time of the killings, she deludedly believed that evil spirits occupied her home, and voices told her that her daughters would painfully die. On 25 September 2003, the day of the killing she saw various supposed omens that she and the girls must die that day. Voices in her head told her 'This is the day you have to do it' (Ellis and Emily, 2006).

Organisational problems

Among organisational problems that can hinder prevention are several which were evident in the cases examined. These are Missed Indications of Accumulating Risk (MIAR), Gaps in Liaison and Information Sharing (GLIS), Weaknesses in Listening to and Questioning Relatives (WLQR), Lack of Overarching Assessments (LOA), Inadequate Physical Safety Precautions (ISP), and Not Recognising Symptoms (NRS). Some of these interrelate, for example 'Lack of Overarching Assessment' can influence 'Missed Indications of Accumulating Risk'.

Missed Indications of Accumulating Risk (MIAR)

These include the individual showing violence, not taking medications, and breaking contact with mental health services. These can happen suddenly and in rapid succession, requiring authorities to be alert and to share information with other services to gain a comprehensive picture. Accumulating risk of violence was evident with Lewis-Ranwell, Nandap, Simelane, Carter, Crook, Dixon, and Diaz. In the cases of Nanadap and Simelane it was accompanied by several other organisational problems.

Gaps in Liaison and Information Sharing (GLIS)

This feature often relates to liaison and information sharing by services, charities, organisations, and others. Within a single organisation there may be different systems of recording that are not compatible or that overlap or have gaps. Such information as there is may not be absorbed by relevant staff either owing to pressures of time or lack of awareness. Across services the potential for missing vital information increases where systems are different and where there may be professional caution in sharing. Issues relating to information sharing and liaison arose with Bobokulova, Nandap, Simelane, Tyler, Carter, and Harris. In Bobokulova's case there were particular challenges because she worked in Russia and she had been treated in a clinic in Ukraine some years previously.

Weaknesses in Listening to and Questioning Relatives (WLQR)

Sometimes authorities are contacted by a relative of a person with SMD who provide information, raise concerns, or report violence to themselves or others. Where this is not clearly recorded, assessed, and acted upon, opportunities for prevention can be missed. Lacey, Nandap, Simelane, Crook, and Bruce provide examples. Sometimes, a general lack of professional inquisitiveness can lead to information and insights being missed. For example, staff failed to enquire why Lacey had attacked his father and half-brother.

Lack of Overarching Assessments (LOA)

Overarching assessment refers to comprehensive evaluation bringing together information including other assessments that have been made over time for a so-called longitudinal assessment. Among other benefits, longitudinal assessments can show the changes that indicate a current acceleration of the risk of violence. It is hindered or assisted by the quality of liaison and information sharing among services. This arose with Lewis-Ranwell, Nandap, Simelane, and Dixon. For example, regarding Nandap, no Merlin report was created so that mental health concerns were not sufficiently highlighted to others.

Inadequate Safety Precautions (ISP)

Occasionally inadequate or lack of safety precautions can allow violence which might otherwise be avoided. These include protective clothing and vehicles for police. As well as physical protection, procedural protection is relevant, such as assessing risks when meeting a patient with SMD and determining the setting, time, and other aspects that can enhance safety. This arose with Bonds in relation to police protection, and with Davydov and Dixon concerning procedures for the personal safety of mental health care workers.

Not Recognising Symptoms (NRS)

Opportunities can be missed where an individual is mis-diagnosed, or assumed to be faking symptoms, or where signs of a SMD are not picked up. This can relate to lack of staff training in recognising the signs of particular mental disorders or features such as psychosis and the potential variety and subtlety of their presentation. This issue arose with Lacey whose presentation was complex and Devanov who was mistakenly thought to be faking mental disorder.

Table 8.1 summarises the features that arose in the cases described earlier in the chapter. The ticks indicate the presence of a feature. Seventeen of the 25 cases described in the glossary are included as these provide material that suggests missed opportunities and consequently strategies for prevention.

Table 8.1 Organisational and related issues in services

MIAR = Missed Indications of Accumulating Risk; GLIS = Gaps in Liaison and Information Sharing; WLQR = Weaknesses in Listening to and Questioning Relatives; LOA = Lack of Overarching Assessments; ISP = Inadequate Physical Safety Precautions; NRS = Not Recognising Symptoms (NRS).						
Name	MIAR	GLIS	WLQR	LOA	ISP	NRS
Lewis-Ranwell	/			/		
Lacey			/			/
Bonds					/	
Bobokulova		/				
Nandap	/	/	/	/		
Simelane	/	/	/	/		
Tyler		/				
Carter	/	/				
Devanov						/
Harris		/				
Crook	/		/			
Davydov					/	
Dixon	/			/	/	
Bruce			/			
Wright	/					
Diaz	/					
Totals	7	6	5	4	3	2

Lack of suitable treatment

Insufficient provision for effective treatment can be an organisational limitation profoundly inhibiting prevention. Where mental disorder has been identified and violence has been perpetrated or a high risk of violence identified, effective treatment can help prevent later violence and homicide. The use of anti-psychotic medication may be part of the treatment plan. Enough psychiatric beds are necessary for the admission of acutely ill patients and funding to allow provision for long enough to allow symptoms to be controlled. A small number of beds will need to be available for severely and chronically ill patients for whom existing medication may not be effective (Torrey, 2012, p. 184).

Among examples of effective out-patient services is the PACT model in the US offering comprehensive locally based treatment to people with serious and persistent mental disorders.

It provides individualised services directly to clients. They receive the 24-hour multidisciplinary staffing of a psychiatric unit within the control of their own home and neighbourhood. PACT team members are trained in psychiatry, social work, nursing, substance abuse, and vocational rehabilitation to meet treatment, rehabilitation, and support needs (e.g. Fresno County, 2020).

Well known is the clubhouse community mental health service model which brings together vocational training, housing, and rehabilitation services and support. Individuals with mental disorders meet to socialise and learn job skills. There may be housing programmes, and contracts with businesses to develop job skills (McKay, Nugent, Johnsen, Eaton, and Lidz, 2016).

Conclusion

Organisation and communication approaches in services and across services interact with each other but can nevertheless be considered under several groupings.

Being alert to a sudden and rapid increase in the risk of homicide or other violence from a potential perpetrator can be preventive. Communicating information within and across services helps ensure that a comprehensive picture is built up. Police may be aware of recent escalating threats and violence while mental health services are more likely to know of an individual's refusal to take medication or attend for treatment.

A precursor to such alertness to escalating risk is that services have systems and personnel that help ensure information is shared effectively. Suitable liaison is built up over time and cannot just be switched on in a crisis. The interface between the community and services is important where members of the public bring their concerns. Procedures for evaluating and acting on such information should be clear.

Related to this is the way that any information, concerns, or reports of a relative of someone with SMD are dealt with. There are instances where relatives have put up red flags which have not been recognised and acted upon and which could have prevented violence.

When relatives are questioned about an incident or about the behaviour of a person with SMD the interview needs to be probing, demonstrating a professional curiosity on the part of the interviewer.

Overarching assessment implies that relevant information from different sources such as services is brought together to inform decision making about an individual with SMD.

Risk assessments for professionals working with individuals having SMD need to take account of protection through physical safeguards like clothing and working vehicles. Procedural protection is relevant such as assessing risks when meeting a patient with SMD. This will include reviews of the proposed setting, time, and other aspects. Such protections need to be conveyed to all relevant staff in a service and supplemented by training and by support, as necessary.

To help ensure that professionals recognise symptoms of SMD, training drawing on the most up to date information and advice in accurate assessment and diagnosis can be provided. This should take account of the subtlety and complexity of some presentations of a condition.

Treatment may include programmes such as PACT and the clubhouse models as used in the US.

Suggested activities

Select a case from the glossary of the book in which organisational constraints appear to have hindered prevention. Use the internet and other references to further explore the events surrounding it. Consider your observations in the light of the issues discussed in the present chapter. Were any further issues pertinent? What other preventive approaches might reduce the risk of homicide?

Key texts

Reed, A. (2014) *Homicide Investigation Report into the Death of a Child* (STEIS Reference 2013/7122) (September 2014) www.birminghamandsoli hullccg.nhs.uk/about-us/publications/safeguarding/527-christina-edkins-hom icide-investigation-report/file.

Jenkins, G. and Moor, N. (2017) *An Independent Investigation into the Care and Treatment of P in the West Midlands.* Niche Health and Social Care Consulting (14 June 2017).

Both of these reports relate to Phillip Simelane's killing of Christina Edkins.

Niche (May 2014) *An Independent Investigation into the Care and Treatment of a Mental Health Service User (MC) in Bristol.* Niche.

This report relates to Marc Carter's killing of Gino Nelmes.

References

Australian Associated Press (2017) 'Mother psychotic when she killed eight children, Queensland court rules' *Guardian* (4 May 2017) www.theguardian.com/australia-news/ 2017/may/04/mother-psychotic-when-she-killed-eight-children-queensland-court-rules.

Barr, C. W., Londoño, E. and Morse, D. (2006) 'Patient admits killing psychiatrist, police say' *Washington Post* (5 September 2006) www.washingtonpost.com/wp-dyn/content/article/2006/09/04/AR2006090400430.html.

BBC News (2003) 'Mother and son killed by "psychotic"' BBC News (15 December 2003) http://news.bbc.co.uk/1/hi/england/beds/bucks/herts/3322525.stm.

BBC News (2013) 'Mental health review after Cray's Hill double death incident' BBC News (27 March 2013) www.bbc.co.uk/news/uk-england-essex-21951670.

BBC News (2015) 'Manslaughter: Timothy Crook guilty of killing parents' BBC News (20 July 2015) www.bbc.co.uk/news/uk-england-wiltshire-33599525.

Bernstein, E. and Koppel. N. (2008) 'A death in the family' *Wall Street Journal* (16 August 2008) www.wsj.com/articles/SB121883750650245525.

Celona, L. and Golding, B (2017) 'NYPD cop-killer was a schizophrenic off his meds: girlfriend' *New York Post* (5 July 2017) https://nypost.com/2017/07/05/nypd-cop-killer-was-a-schizophrenic-off-his-meds-girlfriend/.

Docking, N. (2018) 'Man stabbed his mum to death and tried to kill his gran's carer in psychotic episode' *Echo* (21 December 2018) www.liverpoolecho.co.uk/ news/liverpool-news/christian-lacey-liz-lacey-murder-15584632.

Ellis, T. M. and Emily, J. (2006) 'Child-killer to leave hospital' *The Dallas Morning News* (10 November 2006) www.pressreader.com/usa/the-dallas-morning-news/20061110/281552286359490.

Evans, M. (2018) 'Widow of academic stabbed to death on his doorstep demands to know why psychotic knifeman was released to kill' *Telegraph* (2 July 2018) www.telegraph.co.uk/news/2018/07/02/psychotic-killer-attacked-new-father-told-police-leave-dead/.

Falkenberg, L. (2003) 'Closing arguments begin in Texas mother's murder trial' *Associated Press* (3 April 2003) www.cephas-library.com/assembly_of_god/ assembly_of_god_member_killed _her_sons.html.

Fresno County (2020) *Programme of Assertive Community Treatment (PACT)* https://fresno.networkofcare.org/mh/library/article.aspx?id=311.

Gilligan, A. (2013) 'Truth about dangerous mental patients let out to kill' *The Telegraph* (5 October 2013) www.telegraph.co.uk/news/uknews/crime/10358251/Truth-about-dangerous-mental-patients-let-out-to-kill.html.

Jenkins, G. and Moor, N. (2017) *An Independent Investigation into the Care and Treatment of P in the West Midlands.* Niche Health and Social Care Consulting (14 June 2017).

Joyner, J. (2004) 'Mom cut off baby's arms' *Outside the Beltway* (23 November 2004) www.outsidethebeltway.com/mom_cut_off_babys_arms/.

Lagos, M. (2002) 'Jury finds Attias guilty of murder' *Daily Nexus* (6 June 2002) http://dailynexus.com/2002-06-06/jury-finds-attias-guilty-of-murder/.

McKay, C., Nugent, K. L., Johnsen, M., Eaton, W. W., Lidz, C. W. (2016) 'A systematic review of evidence for the clubhouse model of psychosocial rehabilitation' *Administration and Policy in Mental Health and Mental Health Services Research* 45, 1, 28–47 (31 August 2016).

Milwaukee County Case 2003CF001468 *State of Wisconsin vs. Keith Michael Addy* https://wcca.wicourts.gov/caseDetail.html?cacheId=19D57A47CFCA121AB4538508BF3315A7&caseNo=2003CF001468&countyNo=40&mode=details&offset=11&recordCount=12#summary.

Morris, S. (2019) 'Killer of three elderly Devon men found not guilty of murder due to insanity' *The Guardian* (2 December 2019) www.theguardian.com/uk-news/2019/dec/02/killer-of-three-elderly-devon-men-found-not-guilty-due-to-insanity.

NHS England (2013) *Report to NHS England of the Independent Investigation into the Healthcare and Treatment of 'Patient P'* (Commissioned by the Former North East Strategic Health Authority) http://hundredfamilies.org/wp/wp-content/uploads/2013/12/ RONALD_DIXON_May06.pdf.

Niche (May 2014) *An Independent Investigation into the Care and Treatment of a Mental Health Service User (MC) in Bristol.* Niche.

Reed, A. (2014) *Homicide Investigation Report into the Death of a Child* (STEIS Reference 2013/ 7122) (September 2014) www.birminghamandsolihullccg.nhs.uk/about-us/p ublications/safeguarding/527-christina-edkins-homicide-investigation-report/file.

Reporter (3 April 2006) 'Paranoid schizophrenic Marc Carter jailed for Bristol Samurai sword killing of Gino Nelmes' *HuffPost* (1 February 2013 and updated 3 April 2013) www.huffingtonpost.co.uk/2013/02/01/pranoid-schizophrenic-man2599343.html.

Reporter (2 August 2007) 'Schizophrenic addicted to skunk cannabis killed best friend' *Evening Standard* (2 August 2007) www.standard.co.uk/news/schizophrenic-addic ted-to-skunk-cannabis-killed-best-friend-6602755.html.

Reporter (18 December 2007) 'Jones found not guilty by reason of insanity' *The Connection* (18 December 2007) www.connectionnewspapers.com/ news/2007/ dec/ 18/jones-not-guilty-by-reason-of-insanity/.

Savill, R. (2001) 'Son-in-law stabbed to death in marital bed' *The Telegraph* (6 June 2001) www.telegraph.co.uk/news/uknews/1311615/Son-in-law-stabbed-to-death-in-marital-bed. html.

TASS (2016) 'The murder of a child in Moscow: Investigation progress and public reaction' TASS (29 February 2016) https://tass.ru/proisshestviya/2706157 (in Russian).

Teetor, P. (2002) 'Prelude to a Death' *Los Angeles Times* (5 May 2002) www.latimes. com/archives/la-xpm-2002-may-05-tm-41435-story.html.

Torrey, E. F. (2012) *The Insanity Offense: How America's Failure to Treat the Seriously Mentally Ill Endangers its Citizens.* London, W.W. Norton.

Twomey, J. (2009) 'Fury after psychotic killer walks free after four years' *Express* (22 April 2002) www.express.co.uk/news/uk/96406/Fury-as-psychotic-killer-walks-free-a fter-4-years.

Welton, B. (2013) 'Birmingham bus killer Philip Simelane to be held at a psychiatric unit indefinitely' *Manchester Evening News* (2 October 2013) www.manchester eveningnews.co.uk/news/uk-news/birmingham-bus-killer-phillip-simelane-6128265.

Chapter 9

Retrospect

Introduction

This chapter brings together the themes and findings relating to understanding and preventing homicides by perpetrators with SMD. Regarding understanding, it reviews key aspects of SMD, homicide, and prevention; aspects of Situational Crime Prevention relating to SMD related homicide; and perpetrator and victim demographics and relationships. In relation to prevention, important aspects are: red flags indicating increased risk of violence and potentially homicide; recognising increasing and accumulating risks of violence and possible homicide, and considering psychiatric care as a source of prevention and protection; organisational improvements such as developing better holistic working and communication; and wider issues, for example controlling weapons.

Understanding

Key aspects of understanding SMD, homicide, and prevention

SMD

Underpinning many SMDs is psychosis, characterised by delusions, hallucinations, disorganised speech, grossly disorganised or catatonic behaviour, and negative symptoms. Among SMDs are disorders or aspects of disorders including schizophrenia (sometimes with delusions of persecution), substance/medication-induced psychotic disorder, depressive disorder, and manic episodes.

Schizophrenia, a serious mental disorder affecting how a person thinks, feels, and behaves, is associated with losing touch with reality. It can involve delusions of persecution in which the individual believes that they are being harmed or harassed by another person or organisation.

Substance/medication induced psychotic disorder involves prominent delusions and/or hallucinations owing to the physiological effects of a substance or medication. Psychoactive substances that can cause this disorder include alcohol,

DOI: 10.4324/9781003172727-11

cannabis, inhalants, amphetamines, and cocaine, while among implicated medications are anaesthetics, analgesics, antidepressants, and anticonvulsants.

Depression involves depressed mood and/or great or total diminution of pleasure in activities previously enjoyed. It may be associated with weight change, disturbed sleep, and poor concentration and can significantly impair ability to function at work and socially. Depression also increases suicide risk.

A manic episode can be a symptom of other disorders, including schizoaffective disorder and bipolar disorder. It involves expansive, or irritable mood and goal-directed activity or energy that are abnormally and persistently increased. Symptoms can include an inflated sense of self-esteem or grandiosity, less need for sleep, being more talkative than usual, 'flight of ideas', or racing thoughts, distractibility, higher goal directed activity or psychomotor agitation, and excessive involvement in activities having likely painful consequences.

Homicide

Homicide involves killing another person with varying levels of culpability reflected in different terms including 'degrees' of murder, and manslaughter. In legal proceedings, special defences allow a conviction lesser than murder and include 'diminished responsibility' (impaired mental responsibility). Typologies of homicide often reflect the relationship between perpetrator and victim as with 'matricide'. Means of killing may be indicated such as 'strangling'. Other categorisations include 'murder–suicide', and 'domestic homicide'.

Where a person with SMD perpetrates homicide, they may be judged to have committed manslaughter rather than murder because of 'diminished responsibility'. Also, a defendant may be found to be 'not guilty by reason of insanity' or 'not criminally responsible'. Legal determination of insanity usually relates to tests of criminal responsibility such as the McNaghton Rule.

Prevention and risk reduction

In preventing homicide, the aim is to avoid homicide 'arising', or to stop it happening, implying respectively a longer process or a more immediate intervention. As many homicides are not preventable, it may be more realistic to speak of reducing homicide risk.

Situational Crime Prevention in relation to SMD homicide

SCP and its origins

Situational Crime Prevention (SCP) seeks to reduce crime by analysing the circumstances engendering specific kinds of crime. Recognising that certain situations and settings provide opportunities to commit offences, SCP uses modifications both to the environment and to the management of situations to change how opportunity is structured for the crimes to occur.

SCP was developed by Ron Clarke, a research officer at the Kingswood Training School, Bristol, England, a boarding school for delinquent boys. Clarke examined the situations in which absconding occurred and realised that altering situational features could reduce running away.

Aspects of SCP: theories and behavioural features

Techniques of SCP draw on theories implying that an offender has certain tendencies and acts in particular ways, that individuals behave rationally and make rational choices, that they can act independently, and that they behave hedonistically. SCP takes a behavioural view of people's actions. So-called emotional states are regarded more behaviourally as 'internal dispositions'. SCP can take account of subculture in using preventive techniques in specified circumstances. This requires that the values and beliefs involved are empirically identifiable and can be manipulated to modify decision making in a specific situation.

Preventive interventions that remove opportunities to commit crime

Features of SCP include behavioural approaches and 'scripts' which help researchers to analyse and understand the expectations around certain situations. The location of crime, and products and services can be designed and modified to stop or reduce the occurrence of crime. In developing preventive strategies, practitioners assume that offenders committing crimes make rational choices. Concentrating on specific offences, SCP develops preventive interventions by removing opportunities for the crime to be carried out

SCP strategies and techniques

Five general strategies of SCP are each associated with five opportunity reducing techniques. To increase the effort of perpetrators, strategies include 'target harden' and 'control tools/weapons'. Increasing the risks, includes 'reducing anonymity' and 'strengthening formal surveillance'. Among techniques to reduce rewards to the perpetrator are 'remove targets', and 'deny benefits'. Regarding reducing provocations, techniques include 'reduce frustrations and stress', and 'discourage imitation'. To remove excuses concerns approaches to 'set rules', 'post instructions', 'alert conscience', 'assist compliance' and 'control drugs and alcohol'.

Applying SCP

Several issues are important in applying SCP to homicide perpetrated by individuals with severe mental disorder. They include the predictability of some aspects of psychotic behaviour, 'hard' behavioural interventions, and environmental triggers.

Demographics

Features of perpetrators of homicide with SMD

A sample of homicides between 2000 and 2020, almost all in the UK and the US, were discussed. These involved perpetrators who were evaluated to be not fully responsible for the homicide because of SMD, such as schizophrenia, delusions of persecution, and psychotic episodes. While the small sample size makes generalisations limited, the information can provide an illustration of some features. In line with wider research findings, some perpetrators notably had a history of violence preceding the homicide, sometimes over years, and abused drugs including alcohol. A few declined to take their medication.

Recurrences of illness with individuals having a long history of SMD may seem unexceptional making it hard for professionals to anticipate homicidal violence and requiring careful monitoring. With comparatively sudden onset of SMD, the signs may be missed because unexpected, needing training and vigilance enabling professionals to recognise signs such as psychosis in all its variations.

Perpetrator demographics

Homicide perpetrators with SMD (like perpetrators of homicide generally) tend to be male and aged around 20 to 40 years. US general homicide data indicate an over-representation of black and African American perpetrators. However, perpetrators with SMD were very largely white British and white American reflecting the UK and US wider population demographics. Most perpetrators with SMD of known employment status were unemployed men, seemingly owing to their mental health problems. Seven of the 25 perpetrators killed two or more victims each. Three of these instances were children killed by their mothers.

Victim demographics

Victims of homicide in general are typically young men in their twenties. However, most victims of perpetrators with SMD, were aged 0 to 20 years, and eleven of these were aged 0 to 10 years. Eight victims were aged 61 or over. This higher preponderance of younger and older victims reflects their vulnerability by age. For victims of perpetrators with SMD, the gender balance was roughly equal. By contrast, most perpetrators were aged 21 to 40 years, reflecting their physical strength compared with victims (especially child victims). A similar number of victims were male as were female, unlike perpetrators who were very predominantly male.

In US homicides in general 52.4% of victims were black or African American, and 43.1% were white. In SMD cases, there were no black British or

African American victims. The largest groups were white British and white American, mirroring wider population demographics in the UK and USA. 'Other' ethnic groups were also large and included seven children of Torres Island heritage all killed by one perpetrator. Also in cases of SMD, victim and perpetrator usually had the same ethnicity, perhaps reflecting close ties between members of each ethnic group. In only seven instances did perpetrator and victim differ in ethnic background and of these, five were killings of strangers, none indicating racial or cultural motives. Perpetrators and victims of the same ethnicity were often from one family.

Regarding the social background of victims, the largest group were children including school students (15 of 41) followed by retired people (7 of 41). Relating to the SMD of perpetrators, one victim was a resident in a mental health facility, while two were mental health workers trying to support the perpetrator. Five victims were killed while working. Again, the relatively high proportion of children and school students and of retired people (22 of the 41 victims) indicates the victims that were vulnerable by age. Comparing victims and perpetrators, no victim was unemployed but 13 perpetrators (all male) were, likely owing to mental health problems and sometimes a background of violence. Of perpetrators, four women were home-based parents while only one victim was.

Offender–victim relationships

Concerning general homicides, with male on male homicides, often the participants are acquaintances or strangers after which come friends and family members. However, in male on female killings, over a half the women are victims of intimate femicide. Fewer than 10% are killed by a stranger. Women tend to kill intimate partners or ex-partners and family members (their children).

With most SMD cases, there was a relationship between perpetrator and victim. These were being family members (10), professional and client (4), friends or acquaintances (3), or a former partner (1). In only seven examples were the perpetrator and victim strangers. Multiple victims occurred with family members (4 of 10 cases), friends or acquaintances (1 of 3 cases) and strangers (2 of 7 cases).

Prevention

Identifying and responding to red flags

Among red flags for indicating increased risk of violence and potentially homicide are certain symptoms and aspects of SMD: people with SMD declining to take prescribed medication, substance abuse, a history of violence, and lack of contact with mental health services. Using actuarial instruments and personal interviews in assessing the risk of violence can contribute to prevention.

Recognising symptoms and aspects of SMD associated with violence and homicide

Given the complex nature of SMD, assessment can be challenging, and indications may be missed. Episodic features of some forms and manifestations of schizophrenia are an example. Concerning schizophrenia, an increased potential for violence is associated with delusions of persecution, misidentification, threat, and control; and hallucinations generating negative emotions, and command hallucinations. Symptoms strongly associated with fatal assault are evolving auditory hallucinations and delusional beliefs, convincing the individual that they are endangered. First episode psychotic illness presents the greatest risk of homicide.

Related to these issues are the supposed motives of perpetrators. These may involve command hallucinations, animosity towards the victim or wider group, conviction that the victim threatens the perpetrator, beliefs antipathetic to the victim, general feelings of persecution and threat, and a mission to kill.

Mental health professionals and general physicians need to be able to recognise the symptoms of SMD that are associated with increased risk of violence and seek further specialist advice, as necessary. Other services and facilities that can be alert to mental disorders and to deterioration include police, staff in homeless shelters, social workers, prison personnel, and probation officers. Training drawing on the most up to date information and advice in accurate assessment and diagnosis is required, taking account of the subtlety and complexity of different presentations of conditions.

Where an individual experiences evolving auditory hallucinations and delusional beliefs that convince them that they are endangered, regular monitoring can provide indications of potential violence.

Previous history of violence

A strong indicator of violence is a history of it. This includes having previously been hospitalised for a violent episode, and the main reason for admission to hospital being violence to others (or self-harm). In cases of very recent violence, it is important that any services involved communicate details including information from relatives and friends of the perpetrator to other interested parties.

People with SMD declining to take prescribed medication

Having SMD while declining prescribed medication can be associated with violence including homicide. Individuals with schizophrenia not complying with medication requirements may be more likely to be arrested, re-hospitalised, or commit violent acts.

Non-compliance with medication requirements is more likely if the individual does not recognise that they have SMD (anosognosia). Regular monitoring of individuals who are prescribed medication relating to SMD should help to quickly pick up noncompliance. Discussions can be held with the patient about lack of compliance to see if matters can be rectified. Using long acting medication requiring less frequent administration can be considered.

Substance abuse and the risk of violence

Substance abuse is associated with violence broadly and presents an even higher risk in combination with SMD. For example, where offenders have schizophrenia, major depression, or bipolar disorder, and experience alcohol abuse/dependence this can increase the likelihood of violence and homicide. Certain drugs of themselves can induce psychotic episodes.

Broad responses include better control of illegal drugs and controls on the purchase and consumption of alcohol, although this does not tackle the abuse of readily available substances and home-made drugs.

Lack of contact with mental health services

Sometimes, when violence or homicide has been perpetrated by a person with SMD they have not been in contact with mental health services, reducing the likelihood of prevention. This applies to individuals already known to have SMD, as well as first-timers who, if identified, might have received support. Homicide might be reduced by improving the take up of these services, and by initiatives encouraging individuals with SMD to access mental health support.

Actuarial instruments and personal interviews in assessing the risk of violence

When assessing the risk of violence of individuals with SMD, mental health professionals take account of general risk factors associated with violence, because these may interact with factors associated with SMD, cumulatively increasing risk. Predicting violence from a specific individual with SMD is challenging, because it is infrequent, and its overall prevalence low. Actuarial instruments used in interviewing patients with schizophrenia and assessing risk draw on research suggesting factors associated with increased risk of perpetrating violence. Then the patient is interviewed to uncover unique personal features. Risk factors and unique personal circumstances are both used to help evaluate risk.

Recognising and responding to increasing risk

Indicators of possible increased chances of violence including homicide, such as a history of violence and drug abuse, are not static. They can rapidly become more pronounced or accumulate, so presenting a higher risk. It is important therefore to be alert to any accumulating risk of violence and possible homicide, and to recognise when someone with SMD is exacerbating their condition and the chances of violence. This allows professionals to consider psychiatric care as a source of prevention and protection for the person with SMD and those that they might harm. Where such recognition and treatment has not occurred, it can relate to weak multi professional working and communication.

Recognising accumulating risk of violence and possible homicide

With people with SMD, accumulating signs of risk of violence are not always recognised because they are not seen sufficiently holistically. Observations of people seen by different services are not always communicated across services so that several individuals see part of the picture, but no one sees the whole.

Targeting/prioritising repeat offenders with SMD

Repeat criminals with SMD may be prioritised, for example, by using involuntary commitment to psychiatric care, better guardianship, court-ordered medication, or restraining orders. Targeting those responsible for repeat or chronic disturbances who have SMD has been addressed by police using criminal charges and probation conditions to better control a person's disruptive behaviour, while empowering the community to supervise more effectively.

Recognising that a person with SMD is exacerbating their condition and risk of violence

Sometimes it becomes evident that a person with SMD is by their actions or lack of actions making their condition worse and increasing the chances that they could act violently. Actions may include watching television programmes or seeking out internet sites that feed delusions of persecution such as conspiracy theories, or which depict extreme violence like beheadings. Other actions are taking drugs which may precipitate psychotic episodes and purchasing or otherwise acquiring dangerous weapons such as a sword or a crossbow. Among omissions which can increase the likelihood of violence (and have other deleterious effects) are people declining to take medication

Psychiatric treatment as protection and prevention

It is important that authorities have strategies to improve the take up of mental health services including by acutely psychotic people. These can involve increasing public awareness of such services, working to reduce any stigma associated with them, and monitoring the take up over time to inform further actions.

At the same time, it is necessary for authorities to ensure sufficient treatment for types of SMD associated with increased likelihood of violence. Also needed is provision of intensive care and specialized long-term care to individuals with schizophrenia at high risk for violence. Health authorities need to provide timely psychiatric treatment including, where appropriate, therapy addressing motivational false beliefs.

Where there is an increasing chance of violence and homicide, mental health professionals should be ready to determine (supported by clear policies) whether the individual should be admitted to a residential psychiatric care facility.

Timely effective treatment can help prevent later violence and homicide. This may include prescribing anti-psychotic medication, ensuring enough psychiatric beds for admitting acutely ill patients (with funding for continued provision until symptoms abate) and having a few beds for severely and chronically disordered patients unresponsive to medication.

Outpatient services include the Programme of Assertive Community Treatment (PACT) model in the US offering comprehensive locally based treatment to people with serious and persistent mental disorders. Other interventions include the clubhouse community mental health service model bringing together vocational training, housing, and rehabilitation services and support.

Improving professional and multi-professional working

Weaknesses in professional and multi-professional working and poor communication can lead to missed opportunities to prevent homicide. Preventive responses include developing better holistic working and communication, more rigorously following up concerns of relatives and others, and using agencies while ensuring better supervision of workers with children. Other such responses are developing better supervision and care of residents with SMD in community settings, improving training and understanding of procedures, and protecting mental health professionals.

Developing holistic working and better communication

Service organisation, relationships between services, and lines of communication all influence one another. Professional roles and expectations, and effective communication are crucial for effective multi-professional working.

Being alert to a sudden and rapid increase in the risk of homicide or other violence from a potential perpetrator can be preventive. Police may be aware of recent escalating threats and violence of an individual who has come into their orbit, while mental health professionals are more likely to know of that person's non-compliance with treatment.

Communicating information within and across services can help build a comprehensive picture. But it is not always comprehensive enough. For example, an arresting officer's concerns about an individual may not be passed to an examining physician. Services require well-established systems and trained personnel helping to ensure that vital information is shared effectively.

This interprofessional liaison and information sharing includes health and mental health services, police, social services, staff working in homeless shelters, prison personnel, probation services, and courts.

As well as inter relationships within and between services, the interface between members of the wider community and services is important where members of the public bring their concerns. Procedures for evaluating and acting on such information should be based on clear policy and practice.

Comprehensive assessments of individuals with SMD are useful tools that can help to ensure that relevant information from different sources such as services, relatives, and members of the community are brought together to inform decision making.

Paths for special provision for individuals with SMD

Routes for special provision for people with SMD may be used. Crisis response sites (usually in a hospital) provide streamlined intake procedures and have a no-refusal policy to police, guaranteeing that the individual will at least be evaluated. Jail-based diversion involves redirecting an offender with SMD to treatment rather than prison when the case is reviewed for prosecution, or when it comes to court.

More rigorously following up concerns of relatives and others

Weaknesses sometimes occur in the way that information, concerns, or reports of a relative of someone with SMD are dealt with. Insufficient credence may be placed on concerns of relatives. These may be warnings about an individual's mental condition deteriorating or their taking drugs which are making the condition worse or precipitating psychotic episodes.

When relatives are questioned about an incident or about the behaviour of a person with SMD the interview needs to be probing, reflecting an interviewer's professional curiosity and rigour.

Using agencies and developing better supervision of workers with children

Informal employment practices sometimes lead to unsuitable people being in positions of trust and care. Stricter controls for people working with children can include the wider use of agencies for qualified workers rather than more informal direct employment by parents.

Related to this could be a register of qualified workers, background checks, a requirement for up to date references, and periodic medical and psychological assessments. Overall, this would improve the vetting of people working with those who are vulnerable.

Ensuring better provision for residents with SMD in community settings

Sometimes, residents with mental disorders in a psychiatric setting have been placed at risk by the presence of other residents. For example, in community-based settings such as a 'half-way house' the selection of residents for placement has been in hindsight over-optimistic. Violence including homicide can ensue. This may call for a higher basic level of supervision even in such community-based settings so that staff are more aware of potentially violent situations erupting between residents.

Where there are signs of problems in mental health facilities such as higher rates of people going missing and walking away, management practices, and the physical features and security of facilities can be reviewed and improved, for example through the support of a police liaison officer.

Improving professional training and understanding of procedures

Mental health workers do not always recognise untypical presentations of SMD or enquire into circumstances enough. This suggests retraining in recognising SMD, including the indications of psychosis and in assessing risks, and reminders to properly question the family and carers of mental health patients. Sometimes the custody record needs to be used better and fuller information passed to the examining physician. Overarching reports are sometimes not made (such as Merlin reports in the UK).

To improve the quality of police response, for example, generalist police officers can be better trained to deal with problems involving people with SMD. Generalist police officers with specialist training (and specialist non-police responders) can also be deployed in situations involving individuals with SMD.

Protecting mental health professionals

Risk assessments for professionals working with individuals having SMD need to take account of protection through physical safeguards such as clothing and working vehicles. Procedural protection is relevant such as assessing risks when meeting a client with SMD. This will include reviews of the proposed setting, time, and other aspects. Such protections need to be conveyed to all relevant staff in a service and supplemented by training and support, as necessary.

Professionals should be able to assess the risk of locations and settings and put in place strategies to minimise the chance of violence. This might involve professionals seeing high risk patients with a third-party present and avoiding enclosed spaces. Where workers visit the homes of people with SMD, there should be effective safety procedures translated into practical action and behaviour. Initial training and continuing professional development can highlight better self-protection for mental health workers.

Police on patrol are at risk of violence from criminals and sometimes from people with SMD. Where an officer is attacked in a police vehicle, stronger vehicle protection such as bullet proof windows could be preventive.

Wider issues and related professional responses

Control of weapons

For the general population, including people with SMD, possessing firearms is to some extent curbed by legal controls. Access to firearms is limited, for example, through purchaser background checks and by seizing illegally imported firearms. Risks of the use of edge weapons can be reduced by police stop-and-search powers, confiscating such weapons and prosecuting offenders.

All this applies to people with SMD. Additional measures can include ensuring as far as possible that a person with SMD who is at risk of perpetrating violence does not have access to or possession of obviously dangerous weapons (such as a sword or a crossbow). However, homicides may be perpetrated using beating and bludgeoning, strangulation, driving a vehicle, drowning, and using multiple means, which are clearly much harder to control.

Protection from vehicle attack

To protect pedestrians from random attacks from vehicles, roadside barriers have been erected in busy city areas. Often, the main motivator for this has been terrorist attack, but such steps are preventive more widely.

Chapter 10

Glossary

Around 25 cases (years 2000 to 2020) are listed each with the following information:

Perpetrator = name, age, gender, nationality, race, social background
Victim = name, age, gender, nationality, race, social background
P–V relationship = perpetrator–victim relationship such as 'mother–child' or 'stranger'
Means = weapon or other means involved
Motive = including perpetrator's apparent beliefs and delusions where relevant
Opportunity = including time and date of homicide
Location = place of homicide such as the victim's home or a public place
Preventative strategy = possible foci of prevention
Legal outcome = court judgement on the perpetrator's culpability
Notes = notable further information
References = references for further reading

Alexander Lewis-Ranwell, UK, 2019

Perpetrator	Alexander Lewis-Ranwell, 38, male, white British, AL-R was privately educated. There are no reports of any employment after he left school.
P's mental health	A L-R had been diagnosed with schizophrenia with delusions of persecution.
Victims	Anthony Paine, 80; twins Dick Carter and Roger Carter, 84. All were white British and had retired from working.
P–V relationship	None.
Means	A L-R beat Anthony Paine to death with a hammer, and bludgeoned Dick Carter and Roger Carter with a spade.

DOI: 10.4324/9781003172727-12

Motive	A L-R falsely believed that Anthony Paine was holding a kidnapped girl in his cellar and that the Carter twins were implicated in child abuse and torture.
Opportunity	On 10 February 2019, AL-R having left police custody in Barnstaple, travelled to Exeter were he randomly killed his victims owing to deluded beliefs. He entered the victim's private houses where seemingly no one heard any disturbance.
Location	In Exeter, Anthony Paine was killed in his own house, as were Dick and Roger Carter.
Preventative strategy	Giving greater attention to accumulating indications of risk including in the period shortly before the killings. Potential red flags were AL-R's committing burglary, his threatening a farmer, his mother's worried telephone call to police about her son's release, and police concerns about risk to the public. An overarching assessment could have brought these indications together.
Legal outcome	AL-R was found not guilty by reason of insanity and given a hospital restriction order. The jury raised concerns with the judge about the 'state of psychiatric services' in Devon and the 'failings in care'.
Notes	Devon Partnership and Devon County Council both involved said they would learn lessons.
References	Dilley and Kemp, 2019; Morris, 2019; Sky News, 2019.

Christian Lacey, UK, 2018

Perpetrator	Christian Lacey, 21, male, white British, of no fixed address, seemingly unemployed.
P's mental health	Indications of disturbed behaviour in 2018 included CL's 'disappearance' in London believing that his mobile phone was hacked and that he was going to die, his 25 April attack on his father Johan Wierzbick and his half-brother Jacob Carfoot; his belief that the bathroom towels of the house were evil; and his father finding a hidden knife in CL's bedroom.
Victim	Liz Lacey, 63, female, white British, business adviser for Liverpool Vision. Shortly after killing his mother, CL repeatedly stabbed his grandmother's carer Edwina Holden, 54, who survived.
P-V relationship	Victim Liz Lacey was CL's mother.
Means	Stabbing with a knife.

Motive	Possibly feelings of threat and persecution contributed.
Opportunity	The homicide happened in the early evening of 26 April 2018. Being the victim's son, CL had unchallenged access to her house where he killed her.
Location	At Liz Lacey's home in Hardy Street, Garston, Liverpool.
Preventative strategy	Missed opportunities in 2018 were the 30 March misreading of CL's symptoms at the Royal Liverpool Hospital, and the assessment by Merseycare staff that he did not need to be 'sectioned' into psychiatric care. A case review found that staff failed to enquire why CL had attacked his father and half-brother. Some Criminal Justice Liaison Team members had not received formal training in mental health before joining the team. Police, a physician, and mental health workers may have assumed that CL was not dangerous because of his demeanour. Practitioners did not sufficiently explore CL's complex presentation. Subsequently, Merseycare ordered new training in recognising psychosis and assessing risks, and reminders to employees to properly question the family and carers of mental health patients.
Legal outcome	CL pleaded guilty to the manslaughter of his mother and admitted the attempted murder of carer Edwina Holden. Given an indefinite hospital order, CL was detained at the secure Ashworth Hospital, Maghull.
References	Docking, 2018; Humphries, 2019; Middleton, 2019.

Alexander Bonds, USA, 2017

Perpetrator	Alexander Bonds, 34, male, African American, AB had a criminal background including a 2001 conviction for assaulting a police officer. He was paroled in 2013 for robbery in Syracuse having served nearly seven years of his eight-year sentence. Seemingly unemployed, AB had several aliases, and different addresses including homeless shelters.
P's mental health	It was reported that AB had schizophrenia with delusions of persecution and his girlfriend told investigators that was acting 'irrational and erratic' while off his medication. She claimed that she called emergency services three times on the night of the killing to report AB was 'unhinged' as they walked around the

Bronx. Red flags were AB's previous assault on a police officer and anti-police social media posts although insufficient indication that he would randomly kill an officer.

Victim	Miosotis Familia, 48, female, American Latina, police officer in New York's 46th precinct.
P–V relationship	None, but AB was seemingly hostile to police generally.
Means	The victim was shot to the head with a stolen 0.38 calibre revolver.
Motive	AB apparently hated police indicated by his social media postings.
Opportunity	AB approached a police vehicle in the early hours (12.30 am) of Wednesday 5 July 2017 shooting his victim through the passenger window while she was doing paperwork.
Location	Officer Familia's NYPD vehicle was parked at the corner of Morris Avenue and East 183rd Street New York City.
Preventative strategies	Bullet proof vehicle windows could have been preventive.
Legal outcome	The killing did not come to court as police shot dead the perpetrator fleeing the scene.
References	Celona and Golding, 2017; Cleary, 2017; Hinman, 2018; Prendergast and Sheehan, 2017.

Gyulchekhra Bobokulova Russia 2016

Perpetrator	Gyulchekhra Bobokulova, 38, female, Uzbek national, employed as a nanny.
P's mental health	Years before the killing, GB was treated for schizophrenia.
Victim	Anastasia Meshcheryakova, four years old, female, Russian, had developmental disorder.
P–V relationship	GB was the victim's nanny.
Means	Death was by manual strangulation.
Motive	At the metro station where she was apprehended, GB shouted that she was a terrorist. She told police that she was acting on Allah's orders, and that voices had prompted her to kill Anastasia.
Opportunity	On 29 February 2016 GB remained alone with the victim when parents left their apartment. She strangled the child then severed the head which she took to Oktabrskoye Pole Metro Station in North West Moscow.

Location	Moscow apartment of Vladimir and Ekaterina Mesh-cheryakova the victim's parents.
Preventative strategy	Improvements to the system of registering and subsequently monitoring and supervising workers with vulnerable people.
Legal outcome	GB was charged with murder but evaluated to have schizophrenia, and detained in secure psychiatric hospital.
Notes	GB set fire to the apartment after killing the child.
References	Maynaya, 2016; Reporter 4 March 2016; Reporter 11 March 2016; Reporter 27 April 2016; riafan.ru 29 Feb 2016; TASS 2016.

Timchang Nandap, UK, 2015

Perpetrator	Timchang Nandap, 24, male, Nigerian, black, student possibly at the London University School of Oriental and African Studies, diagnosed with schizophrenia with delusions of persecution.
P's mental health	Signs of TN's deteriorating mental health in the six months prior to the killing were his May 2015 arrest wielding a knife on a London street, high cannabis use, experiencing delusions of persecution and hallucinations; strange behaviour noticed by arresting officers; and his requiring clinical treatment in Nigeria for psychosis including hallucinations.
Victim	Jeroen Ensink, 41, male, Dutch, white, water engineer and academic at London School of Hygiene and Tropical Medicine.
P–V relationship	None.
Means	Stabbing with a knife.
Motive	At the time of the attack TN experienced cannabis induced psychosis.
Opportunity	On the early afternoon 29 December 2015 TN saw Ensink alone and unsuspecting outside the victim's home. Although there were residents in nearby houses when help came Ensink was already dying.
Location	Outside victim's London house in Islington, London.
Preventative strategy	Earlier identification of the accumulating potential risk around TN and the creation of a Merlin report which may have led to TN being treated in psychiatric provision.
Legal outcome	TN, admitting manslaughter on the grounds of diminished responsibility was sentenced to an indefinite hospital order at Broadmoor secure hospital.

Notes	Risk indicators included TN's May 2015 arrest wielding a knife on a London street where his sister lived, sister Wupya Nandap's call to police saying that TN's high cannabis use and watching conspiracy theories on television were worsening his condition, and her warning that he was experiencing 'paranoia' and hallucinations and should not be interviewed alone; arresting officers noticing TN behaving strangely possibly owing to drug abuse or mental illness; a doctor examining TN before the interview claiming that he was given no 'markers' on TN's mental health; seemingly missed information on the custody record; TN answering strangely when interviewed; no Merlin report created on TN so mental health concerns not highlighted to others; TN's clinical treatment in Nigeria for psychosis including hallucinations.
References	Baker, 2018; BBC News, 2018; Davies, 2018a; Davies, 2018b; Evans, 2018.

Raina Thaiday, Australia, 2014

Perpetrator	Raina Mersane Ina Thaiday (aka Mersane Warria), 37, female, Australian, a home-based parent.
P's mental health	RT apparently developed schizophrenia triggered by long-term cannabis use. She became obsessed with hygiene, emptying the house of furniture to clean it and leaving her family to sleep outside on a mattress. She believed that she was 'the chosen one'. Around ten days before the killing, neighbours heard RT on her phone or talking to herself saying strange things like 'I have the power to kill people'.
Victims	RT's three sons, four daughters and a niece aged 2 to 14. Malili Warria (14), Angelina Thaiday (14), Shantae Warria (11), Rayden Warria (9), Azariah Willie (8), Daniel Willie (6), Rodney Willie (5), and Patrenella Willie (2). The family apparently were from Erub Island in the Torres Strait (part of the Torres Strait Islander, Aboriginal and South Sea Islander Communities).
P–V relationship	Seven victims were RT's own children, the eighth was her niece.
Means	RT fatally stabbed the children then stabbed herself repeatedly but survived. Her adult son Lewis Warria, finding RT on the house veranda, summoned police.

Motive	Psychiatrists considered that long term cannabis use triggered RT's schizophrenia. RT believed that she heard a bird call signalling the end of the world and killed the children to save them.
Opportunity	Investigators estimate that the killings occurred between the night of Thursday 18 and the morning of Friday 19 December 2014. RT was the sole adult with the victims who were vulnerable by age.
Location	RT's home, Murray Street, Manoora, Cairns, Australia.
Preventative strategy	Prevention may have been possible if signs of RT's declining mental health had been reported to authorities and acted on. Several psychiatrists testified that RT's mental state likely declined in the months before the killings. Neighbours reported strange behaviour ten days before the killings. However, previously RT had never been treated for mental disorder.
Legal outcome	The court judged RT of unsound mind at the time of the killings and she did not stand trial. She was held in a high security mental health centre in Brisbane.
Notes	After the killing RT was taken to Cairns base hospital under guard and charged with murder next day.
References	ABC News, 2014; BBC News, 2017; Australian Associated Press, 2017.

Phillip Simelane, UK 2012

Perpetrator	Phillip Simelane from Walsall, West Midlands, England, 23 years old, male; Black British. He had previously been in prison. PS was apparently unemployed.
P's mental health	PS began having mental health problems in his mid-teens when he gained several criminal convictions including two offences involving knives. A former patient of the Birmingham and Solihull Mental Health NHS Trust, he was discharged in December 2012 (three months before the killing). PS reportedly had schizophrenia with delusions of persecution.
Victim	Christina Edkins, 16 years old, female; white British, schoolgirl.
P–V relationship	None.
Means	Stabbing in the chest with a knife.
Motive	In court, the judge stated that PS's mental function was 'wholly abnormal' owing to his mental illness leading him to kill Christina because in his deluded state he thought she was a danger to him.

Opportunity	At about 7.30 am on 7 March 2013, PS disembarking a public bus fatally stabbed the victim. Edkins was unsuspecting, PS had a legitimate reason to pass her, and the passengers did not realise immediately what happened.
Location	Public bus in Birmingham, England on which the victim was going to school. PS was later arrested nearby.
Preventive strategy	Ensuring that patients have a care plan, and related treatment and monitoring before being released into the community may have been preventive.
Legal outcome	PS pleaded not guilty on the grounds of diminished responsibility and was sentenced to indefinite hospital detention. The judge expressed concern that PS was not receiving treatment at the time of the killing.
Note	Birmingham and Solihull Mental Health NHS Trust was criticised following the killing. A homicide investigation report was completed in 2014.
References	Bhogal, 2017; Gilligan, 2013; Reed, 2014; Reporter, 2 October 2013; Welton, 2013.

Mark Tyler, UK, 2012

Perpetrator	Mark Tyler, 37, male, white British, married with children, he was known to police, probation, mental health, and drug support services. MT (and his ex-wife) were placed into residential rehabilitation units in 2006 and their four children taken into foster care. In 2010 MT was convicted of firearms and drug offences. He was seemingly unemployed.
P's mental health	Between February 2011 and July 2012 MT had four mental health assessments but no specific condition was diagnosed.
Victim	Maureen Tyler, 79, female, white British. Retired, she previously worked in a local shop at Crays Hill, Basildon, Essex.
P–V relationship	MT was the victim's son.
Means	The victim was killed by a single shot from a sawn-off shotgun.
Motive	MT had a history of drug use which may have contributed to his actions.
Opportunity	The bodies of MT and his mother were found 3 September 2012 after a neighbour called police having not seen them for several days. Maureen Tyler was

likely shot on 27 or 28 August and MT shot himself on 1 September 2012. MT possessed a shotgun, was alone and undisturbed with his mother for several days.

Location	Maureen Tyler's home in Pitsea View Road, Cray's Hill, Basildon, Essex. Maureen Tyler's body was on the living room sofa. MT's body was in the bathroom.
Preventative strategy	Earlier identification of possible psychosis. In July 2012, MT attended a health assessment/psychiatric consultation, but seemingly no diagnosis was made. The health authority was the South Essex Partnership University NHS Foundation Trust. Two investigations followed the deaths.
Legal outcome	A coroner's inquest was held at Essex and Thurrock following the deaths.
Notes	A domestic homicide review by Basildon Community Safety published in November 2015 found that MT took heroin including in 2011 when his father was ill. He exhibited bizarre behaviour. His mother resisted family members' attempts to take MT to hospital, believing she could care for him. The report recommended developing better information sharing and a more multi-agency approach to provide comprehensive support.
References	BBC, 2013; Heart Radio, no date; Nolan, 2013; Porter, 2015.

Marc Carter, UK, 2012

Perpetrator	Marc Carter, 46, male, white British.
P's mental health	MC Diagnosed with schizophrenia with delusions of persecution. A former inpatient of Fromeside secure hospital, he moved to a mental health 'half-way house' days before killing.
Victim	Gino Nelmes, 32, male, white British, adopted as a child, had mental health problems, had a partner and two young children.
P–V relationship	MC and Gino Nelmes were residents at a supported housing property in Filton Avenue, Bristol run by Keystones Mental Health Support Services.
Means	MC stabbed the victim 18 times with a Samurai sword including through the heart, liver and spleen.
Motive	MC seemingly believed that Nelmes was reading his thoughts and repeating them.

Opportunity	Saturday 17 March 2005 when MC and Nelmes were residents at Filton Avenue, Bristol which was supervised during the week but less so at the weekend when the attack took place. MC stabbed Nelmes then reported to Trinity Road police station in another part of the city and confessed.
Location	A 'half-way house' in Filton Avenue, Bristol.
Preventative strategy	Full weekend supervision at the half-way house could have been preventive. Avon and Wiltshire Health Authority opened an investigation and committed to work with an independent investigation designed 'to learn any lessons'.
Legal outcome	April 2006 MC pleaded guilty to manslaughter on the grounds of diminished responsibility. He was ordered to be detained at Broadmoor secure hospital indefinitely with a minimum of 12 years before being eligible for release.
Notes	In March 2012 MC had schizophrenia identified which may have contributed to the killing. MC was considered suitable for a trial release into the community despite a 20-year history of assaults and wounding, convictions for attacks and assaults, and having served nine-year prison sentence.
References	Reporter, 3 April 2006; Reporter, 18 September 2012; Robinson, 2013.

Deyan Devanov, Canary Islands, 2011

Perpetrator	Deyan Devanov, 29, male, Bulgarian who had emigrated to UK. A 'drifter' he had stayed previously in Edinburgh, Ibiza, and North Wales; at the time of the killing he was living in a derelict building on Los Christianos beach, Tenerife (Spanish Canary Islands).
P's mental health	DD was 'sectioned' at his family's request as an involuntary inpatient at a mental health unit Glan Clwyd Ablett Unit, at Ysyty Glan Clwyd, in Bodelwyddan, North Wales. A Health Inspectorate of Wales enquiry report of November 2014 found that DD was misdiagnosed as faking mental illness before his release from the unit in October 2010. DD believed he was Jesus Christ sent to create a new Jerusalem, and heard voices commanding him to kill.

Victim	Jennifer Mills-Westley, 60 years old, female, white British, grandmother. A former road safety officer, she had retired to Tenerife in 2009.
P–V relationship	None.
Means	Beheading with a knife.
Motive	DD may have acted on command hallucinations of voices telling him to kill. He seemingly took drugs.
Opportunity	The homicide took place 13 May 2011 when DD was armed with a knife, and the suspect and others around were unsuspecting.
Location	Mas Articulos Precios shop in the resort of Los Christianos, Tenerife.
Preventive strategy	Better diagnosis before his release from the Ablett psychiatric unit at Ysbyty Glan Clwyd in Bod-elwyddan, North Wales.
Legal outcome	Deyan Devanov was sentenced to 20 years in a secure psychiatric unit on Tenerife.
References	Gilligan, 2013; North Wales Live, 2013; Sky News, 2013.

Michael Harris, UK, 2007

Perpetrator	Michael Harris, 24, male, white British. Reports were unclear about his social background and employment status.
P's mental health	MH had schizophrenia and was prone to violent out-bursts. He smoked skunk cannabis heavily exacerbat-ing his schizophrenia.
Victim	Carl James, 21, male, white British. He lived with his girlfriend Emma Lewis and their daughter Daniella aged three in Park North, Swindon. Reports are unclear about his social background and employment status.
P–V relationship	MH was a long-term friend of the victim.
Means	Stabbing with a knife.
Motive	MH smoked skunk cannabis heavily, possibly exacer-bating his schizophrenia.
Opportunity	On 4 March 2007 MH went unsuspected to his friend's home armed with a knife and killed the victim as he came to the door.
Location	The doorstep of Carl James' home, Swindon, Wilt-shire, England.
Preventative strategy	A report commissioned by the Strategic Health Authority criticised the Avon and Wiltshire Partnership NHS Trust. It found 'an accumulation of poor practice', 'failures in systems', and a lack of 'managerial direction

	and control'. These were causal factors in the victim's death. Better drug control of the use of skunk cannabis could have been preventive.
Legal outcome	At the trial, defence lawyers stated that mental health workers though aware of MH problems failed to intervene. Admitting manslaughter on the grounds of diminished responsibility, MH was held indefinitely under the Mental Health Act at Fromeside Unit a secure mental health unit, Blackberry Hill Hospital, Fishponds, Bristol.
Notes	After killing Carl James, MH walked to his own mother's house, confessed, and awaited police.
References	BBC News, 22 November 2011; Reporter, 2 August 2007; Wiles, 2013.

Timothy Crook, UK, 2007

Perpetrator	Timothy Crook, 51, male, White British, ex-Ministry of Defence worker, made redundant soon after being convicted of harassment against a female work colleague. He was unemployed.
P.'s mental health	TC was 'sectioned' in 2002 and diagnosed with schizophrenia with delusions of persecution. On discharge, he lived with his parents who had difficulty coping with him. He refused contact with mental health services and declined prescribed taking medication.
Victims	Robert Crook, 90, male, white British, retired; Elsie Crook, 83, female, white British, retired.
P–V relationship	The victims were TC's mother and father.
Means	TC kicked, punched, and stamped on the two victims, hit them with a hammer and strangled them with a belt.
Motive	TC at some point believed that police were conspiring against him and US forces were pursuing him. His exact motive for killing is unclear.
Opportunity	TC apparently killed his parents in the late afternoon of Saturday 6 July 2007. He occupied the same house as his parents, who were very elderly, and was uninterrupted.
Location	At the home that RC shared with his parents in Swindon, Wiltshire, England.
Preventative strategy	Approaches to ensure compliance with taking medication and contact with mental health services. Prior to the killing, TC's sister Janice Lawrence claims that she contacted Avon and Wiltshire Mental Health Trust to alert them to concerns about TC.

Legal outcome	After the killing, TC was considered unfit to stand trial because of his mental health problems. Eight years later in 2015, he was found guilty of manslaughter on the grounds of diminished responsibility and detained for life in Rampton Hospital, England.
Notes	After killing his parents, TC drove the bodies 150 miles away to Lincoln, depositing them in the overgrown land of a house he owned. Leaving his car in the area, he caught three trains back to Swindon, Wiltshire, England. On 11 July 2007 the bodies were discovered after police were alerted.
References	BBC News, 2015; Ferris, 2015.

Vitali Davydov, US, 2006

Perpetrator	Vitali Davydov, 19, male, North Potomac, white American; graduated high school in 2005. Having worked for company that trained lifeguards, at the time of the killing was seemingly unemployed.
P's mental health	VD was being treated for schizophrenia and was not taking his medication.
Victim	Wayne Fenton, 53, male, Rockville, Maryland, USA; white American, psychiatrist with a private practice in Bethesda, Maryland.
P–V relationship	VD was Wayne Fenton's patient.
Means	VD beat the victim to death with his fists.
Motive	There may have been an altercation about VD taking his medication.
Opportunity	On Saturday, 2 September 2006, Fenton saw VD in consultation, with VD's father present. An appointment for treatment was made for later that week. On Sunday, 3 September, the patient's father called Fenton, asking him to immediately see VD who was angry about taking medication. At 4 pm, Fenton saw the patient in a small, office behind a locked door, the father having left on an errand. Fenton encouraged VD to take an antipsychotic drug. When the father returned, his son was outside with blood stained hands. Dr Fenton was discovered seemingly dead. VD's father called emergency services, but Fenton was declared dead at the scene. VD told police that he feared a sexual assault.
Location	Psychiatrist's office in Bethesda, Maryland, USA.

Preventative strategy — The Psychiatric Times noted of the case that before accepting patients for consultation or referral for treatment, psychiatrists should inquire about 'the nature and severity of illness, a history of violence, drug abuse, and treatment adherence'. Risk of violence to the clinician increases when severely ill, psychotic patients are seen alone, especially at evenings or on weekends. Clinicians should recognise patients' escalating violence, such as agitation and threats and should have a reliable third party present for the initial evaluation of an unknown patient with SMD.

Legal outcome — In 2007, VD was found guilty but not criminally responsible for the murder of Wayne Fenton and moved to maximum-security psychiatric hospital until considered no longer dangerous.

References — Barr, Londoño and Morse, 2006; Simon, 2011; Wiggin, 2011.

Ronald Dixon, UK, 2006

Perpetrator — Ronald Dixon, 35, male, white British. RD was seemingly unemployed and supported by a mental health charity.

P's mental health — RD first visited his physician with mental health concerns in 1993. A year later, he attacked his parents with a hammer. In January 1997, his parents told police that RD claimed there were spirits in his head. Between September 1997 and March 1998, he was frequently arrested, often claiming he was the Queen's son. From June 1998, to November 1999 RD, detained in psychiatric care, claimed palace doctors performed a lobectomy on him, and the Queen had had a plate inserted into his head displaying his thoughts on a screen. He was diagnosed with symptoms of schizophrenia and 'mania'. In January 2006 RD he was arrested outside Buckingham Palace saying he would kill the Queen.

Victim — Ashleigh Ewing, 22, female, white British, employee of the charity Mental Health Matters.

P–V relationship — The victim, known to RD, worked for a mental health charity and delivered a letter to him at his home.

Means — Repeated stabbing with knives.

Motive — RD seemingly resented receiving a letter about debts he owed a mental health charity.

Opportunity	The homicide occurred on 19 May 2006 when RD was in his own home with knives available and was visited by a lone female mental health worker.
Location	RD's home in Heaton, Newcastle, England.
Preventative strategy	A report criticised staff actions at the Northumberland Tyne and Wear NHS Foundation Trust. A 13 December 2005 review by a consultant and a community psychiatric nurse missed the opportunity to increase monitoring of RD and to clarify inter agency roles. It was recorded that RD risked relapse, having stopped taking medication. RD was arrested in January 2006 in London, returned to Newcastle, and held in a secure unit but not assessed while showing psychotic symptoms. A risk assessment of 13 February 2006 found RD to have 'no apparent risk of ... violence to others'. He was discharged soon afterwards to supported accommodation. By May 16, 2006, there was a 'compelling need' for a community psychiatric nurse to formally review his care following 'significant changes' in RD's presentation. In February 2010 Mental Health Matters admitted failing to protect the victim.
Legal outcome	In court, on October 2007, RD admitting manslaughter on the grounds of diminished responsibility was detained indefinitely at the secure Rampton Hospital, England.
References	NHS England, 2013; Scott, 2013.

William Bruce, USA, 2006

Perpetrator	William Bruce, 23, male, white American, had previously joined the armed forces but had been discharged, and was apparently unemployed.
P's mental health	WB was diagnosed with 'paranoid schizophrenia' (schizophrenia with delusions of persecution) in 2005 after several violent incidents.
Victim	Amy Bruce, 47, female, white American.
P–V relationship	Amy Bruce was WB's mother.
Means	WB hit the victim with a hatchet as she worked at her desk and deposited her body in the bathtub. He was later arrested at his grandfather's house in South Portland.
Motive	WB killed his mother deludedly believing she was an al Qaeda agent.

Opportunity	The homicide occurred on 20 June 2006 when WB was alone in the house with his mother and she was at her desk.
Location	The killing occurred at the victim's home, Caratunk, Maine, USA. Husband Joe Bruce discovered Amy Bruce's body on returning home from work on the afternoon of 20 June 2006.
Preventative strategy	WB's father believed that his son should not have been released from Riverview Psychiatric Recovery Center in April 2006 and blamed patient advocates for pressing for WB's release.
Legal outcome	In 2007, WB was found not guilty of murder by reason of insanity and sent to Riverview Psychiatric Recovery Center, Augusta, Maine. Transferred to a group home in March 2014, WB was returned to Riverview in January 2015 after using illegal drugs.
Notes	WB's pattern of schizophrenia included a 2005 near-fatal hunting accident when he turned a gun on his father and two friends following which he was admitted to Acadia Hospital, Bangor, Maine. He was sent there in 2006 after again attacking his father and on 6 February 2006 was moved to Riverview Psychiatric Recovery Center, Augusta. He was discharged on 20 April 2006, two months before killing his mother.
References	Boston News, 2006; Bernstein and Koppel, 2008; Novacic, 2015.

Nathan Philip Jones, USA, 2006

Perpetrator	Nathan Jones, 26, male, white American, lived with his mother, a former student of the College of William and Mary. Reports are unclear about his social background and employment status.
P's mental health	NJ's father testified in court about his son's declining mental health and not taking his prescribed medication at the time of the killing.
Victim	Pamela Ann Jones, 57, female, white American born in Sydney, Australia who came to US in her twenties to attend nursing school.
P–V relationship	The victim was NJ's mother.
Means	Stabbing. Two bloody knives were found at the scene.
Motive	On the day of the killing NJ seemingly developed psychotic behaviour and his mother was concerned. Placed in seclusion following his arrest, NJ began

	drinking his urine, and eating and smearing himself with his faeces.
Opportunity	On 12 May 2006 NJ was alone in the house where he lived with his mother.
Location	The killing occurred inside the home of Pamela Ann Jones at Mosby Woods, Sherman Street, City of Fairfax. Police found blood in the basement, kitchen, and bathroom of the home, a mop and bucket of bloody water and two blood stained knives.
Preventative strategy	Prevention may have been possible if parents or others had alerted mental health services about NJ's psychotic behaviour and refusal to take medication on the day of the killing.
Legal outcome	In December 2007 the Fairfax County Circuit Court found NJ not guilty of murder by reason of insanity and committed him to psychiatric care.
Notes	Around 4 am on 12 May 2006, Pamela Jones called her estranged husband Dennis Jones saying NJ was acting psychotic. About 7 am Dennis Jones called in and drove NJ to a nearby park to play basketball, telling NJ to take his medication on returning home. Later after being contacted by NJ speaking incoherently, his concerned father picked NJ up in the Fairfax Circle area and started driving home. On the way, NJ became aggressive and declined to go to the house. Denis Jones concerned about Pamela's safety left NJ to drive to her house, finding her body on the bathroom floor.
References	Reporter, 16 May 2007; Reporter, 18 December 2007.

Dena Schloser, USA, 2004

Perpetrator	Dena Schloser, 35, female, white American, mother of three children and a home-based parent.
P's mental health	DS had a history of postpartum depression and seemingly had psychotic episodes. In January 2004, officials were called to DS's home after she was seen running down the street, with one of her daughters bicycling after her. The child told officials her mother had left her six-day-old sister alone in the apartment. DS, apparently suffering from postpartum depression and having a psychotic episode, was hospitalized. She later underwent counselling. Texas Child Protective Services closed a seven-month investigation concluding

	that DS pose no risk to her children. Neighbours regarded DS as a loving mother.
Victim	Margaret Schloser, DS's baby daughter, 11 months, female, white American.
P–V relationship	DS was the victim's mother.
Means	DS amputated the arms of Margaret who was pronounced dead at hospital.
Motive	DS motive seemingly implicated postpartum depression and psychotic episodes.
Opportunity	DS killed Margaret on 22 November 2004 while alone in the house with her. John Schlosser, her husband was at work and her two older daughters aged six and nine were at school.
Location	Alerted by 911 services, police arrived at DS apartment in Plano, Dallas, Texas. They found the baby fatally injured in crib. DS covered in blood was in the living room.
Preventative strategy	There was no family history of violence. Longer treatment for post-partum depression and seeming psychosis might have been preventive.
Legal outcome	Charged with capital murder DS was found not guilty by reason of insanity and placed in psychiatric care. In November 2008 DS was moved from Rusk State Hospital to out-patient care with conditions.
Notes	On the day of the killing DS husband telephoned a day-care centre asking them to check on his wife and daughter. Day-care workers telephoned DS then called emergency services. The 911 service called DS who told them that she had killed her baby.
References	Associated Press, 23 November 2004, 4 January 2015; Joyner, 2004; Religion News Blog, 2008.

Gregory Davis, UK, 2003

Perpetrator	Gregory Davis, 24, male, white British. An arts graduate of Northampton University, later a supermarket supervisor.
P's mental health	In 2003 at the time of the killing GD was diagnosed with depression, alcohol dependence, and social anxiety. GD's 2003 diary stated, 'Quit job tomorrow. Get Mick killed. Get Stuart to withdraw cash every day. When all gone, kill him. Repeat Mick plan ad infinitum all over country and world in Las Vegas and swanky bars'.

Victims	Dorothy Rogers, 48, and her son Michael Rogers, 19, both white British. Their employment status is unclear from reports.
P–V relationship	GD knew divorcee Dorothy Rogers and her partner Michael Cowells from the Pilgrim's Bottle Public House.
Means	In the events surrounding the killing, GD first assaulted Michael Cowells, Dorothy Rogers' partner. He then repeatedly stabbed Dorothy Rogers and stabbed and disembowelled her son Michael Rogers.
Motive	GD kept a diary setting out plans to be a serial killer.
Opportunity	On 28 January 2003, intending to kill Michael Cowells, GD took a knife and a hammer to Dorothy Rogers' home. Following an argument, GD fractured Michael Cowells' skull with the hammer then fatally stabbed Dorothy Rogers, witnessed by her son. Michael Rogers fled the house and GD chased him to a nearby children's playground and fatally stabbed him.
Location	The Rogers' home on the Stantonbury Estate, Great Linford, Milton Keynes, and a nearby children's playground.
Preventative strategy	It might have been preventive if someone had discovered GD's fantasies about becoming a serial killer and reported them.
Legal outcome	In 2003, GD was sentenced to be detained indefinitely in Broadmoor Hospital, Berkshire.
Notes	GD was moved to a less secure hospital in Oxford in 2009.
References	BBC News, 15 December 2003; BBC News, 24 August 2011.

Percy Wright, UK, 2003

Perpetrator	Percy Wright, 35, male, black British, unemployed.
P's mental health	By July 2004 PW's physician found him to be 'anxious and paranoid' and referred him to a hospital mental health unit which he attended twice. No major mental health issue was diagnosed. By January 2005, PW's behaviour had deteriorated, and Colette Lynch warned PW's doctor that he was becoming 'paranoid and aggressive'. Later that day, PW told his doctor that he was hearing voices and that he could change the weather by changing his clothes.

Victim	Colette Lynch, 20, female, nationality, white British, mother of three children: Joshua, 5, Iyesha, 2, and Tia, 1.
P–V relationship	PW was a former partner of Colette Lynch.
Means	PW non-fatally attacked Colette's mother, 58, who was staying with her daughter, then chased Colette Lynch into the street stabbing her with a knife.
Motive	PW's motive appears related to his declining mental health.
Opportunity	The homicide occurred on 3 February 2005. PW had access to Colette's house, having broken in earlier threatening to cut Colette's throat and was armed. With Colette in the house were only her children and her mother so no one could intervene.
Location	At the victim's home in Rugby, Warwickshire, England. PW attacked Colette's mother who was staying there, then chased Colette into the street and killed her.
Preventative strategy	The Independent Police Commission criticised Warwickshire Police for their response to PW's threats of 1 February 2005. Officers failed to arrest PW or record the incident as a crime and did not treat the incident according to their domestic violence policy.
Legal outcome	Admitting manslaughter on the grounds of diminished responsibility, PW was detained in a Bristol psychiatric hospital.
Notes	On 1 February Colette informed the unit that PW had threatened to kill her brother. Hours later, he forced his way into her home, attacked her and threatened to cut her throat but she escaped. At 11.30 pm nurse Samantha Grey telephoned police saying that PW had left hospital (after treatment for injuries sustained breaking into the house) and that his mental health was getting worse. She called police again saying that PW may cause a threat to Colette. Police were sent but were diverted to another incident before they found PW. Next night PW was assessed by a social worker outside his house to be fit to remain there. Before a planned formal assessment could be carried out, PW killed Colette.
References	Dolan, 2009; Twomey, 2009.

Lisa Ann Diaz, USA, 2003

Perpetrator	Lisa Ann Diaz, 24, female, American Latina. LAD experienced a chaotic, emotionally deprived childhood. At 17 she had a daughter (Misty) by David Sanchez

whom she later married. They divorced in 1996. Next year, LAD married Angel Diaz, a quality control manager whom she met at their Dallas workplace. They had two daughters Briana and Kamryn After 2000, LAD became a home-based parent.

P's mental health From 2002, Lisa reported experiencing many ailments, making numerous visits to doctors or alternative therapists. She developed an obsessive fear of germs, believing that she had transmitted her illnesses to her children. On 2 September 2003, LAD saw Dr Wilkinson, who suggested her problems were psychosomatic and referred her to Dallas psychiatrist. LAD did not attend.

Victims LAD's daughters Kamryn aged three and Briana aged five.

P–V relationship LAD was the victims' mother.

Means LAD drowned the children in a bathtub.

Motive LAD deludedly believed that evil spirits occupied her home, and voices told her that her daughters would painfully die. On the day of the killing she saw various supposed omens (such as crows on the lawn) that she and the girls must die that day. Voices in her head told her 'This is the day you have to do it'.

Opportunity The homicides occurred on the afternoon of 25 September 2003. Opportunity arose because LAD was responsible for the children and her husband was at work. She drove Briana to kindergarten and took Misty to school. At 2: 45 p.m., LAD brought Briana home from school. LAD drew water in the bathroom tub for Briana, said a prayer and drowned her. LAD then drowned Kamryn. Placing the bodies on her bed, LAD, stripped, entered the shower, and repeatedly stabbed herself with a kitchen knife.

Location LAD's apartment, Plano, Texas.

Preventative strategy Earlier intervention as LAD's mental health deteriorated.

Legal outcome Tried in 2004 LAD was found not guilty by reason of insanity and admitted to Big Spring State Hospital, Texas.

Notes LAD told her husband on his return from work at 6.35 pm that 'something happened to the girls'. He discovered their bodies in the bedroom.

References Ellis and Emily, 2006; Whitley, 2005.

Deana Laney, USA 2003

Perpetrator	Deana Laney, 39, female, white American. DL home schooled her children.
P's mental health	DL was a member of an Assemblies of God church. A year before killing her children she told church members that the world was ending, and that God had ordered her to get her house in order.
Victims	DL's sons Joshua, eight, and Luke, six. Also attempted to kill her son Aaron aged 14 months.
P–V relationship	DL was the victims' mother.
Means	Beaten on the head by a rock. After the killing DL telephoned emergency services at midnight and told them she had killed the boys.
Motive	DL claimed that God told her to kill her sons.
Opportunity	The killings took place on the night of Friday 9 May 2003 (Mothers' Day weekend). DL killed the children outside while her husband slept in the house then alerted emergency services.
Location	The yard of her home in New Chapel Hill, near Tyler, Texas. Deputies arrived at 12:52 am Saturday 10 May. Entering the house, they found Aaron in his crib wounded but still breathing. In woods behind her house, DL told officers where her other two children could be found. Her husband emerged apparently roused from asleep.
Preventative strategy	No preventive strategies are apparent. Neighbours believed that the Laney family appeared to be stable and loving and DL had no history of mental disorder.
Legal outcome	DL seemingly had psychotic delusions at the time of the killing making her unable to distinguish right and wrong. In 2004 the Smith County court found her not guilty by reason of insanity. DL was committed to Kerrville State Hospital from 2004 to May 2012. She was then released subject to conditions, including having no unsupervised contact with minors and regular tests to ensure compliance with taking medication.
References	CNN/KLTV, 2003; Falkenberg, 2003.

Keith Michael Addy USA, 2003

Perpetrator	Keith Michael Addy, 26, male, white American, a former sex offender. Reports are unclear about his social background and employment status.

P's mental health	KMA may have experienced an unrecognised mental disorder for a year before killing.
Victim	Annamarie Lewandowski, 19, female, white American, Worked for 'Beautiful Blondes' an escort service, mother of a one-year-old baby.
P–V relationship	KMA did not know the victim before she visited his apartment as an escort service employee.
Means	KMA hit the victim with a hammer and stabbed her before dismembering her body.
Motive	MKA told detectives that voices ordered him to kill Lewandowski and that he was possessed by demons.
Opportunity	The homicide occurred Thursday 6 March 2003. KMA was alone and uninterrupted in his own apartment with the escort.
Location	KMA's apartment in 8700 block of W. National Avenue, West Allis, Milwaukee County, Wisconsin.
Preventative strategy	KMA reportedly had an unnoticed mental disorder the year before the killing.
Legal outcome	Found not guilty by reason of mental disease or defect, KMA was committed for psychiatric treatment at the State Mental Institution, Madison, Wisconsin.
Notes	In March 2003, when Lewandowski visited MKA's apartment as an escort he covered her head with a hood and tied her up. He dripped hot wax on her, repeatedly hit her over the head with a framing hammer, and finally repeatedly stabbed her. An hour later he dismembered her body with a saw in the bathtub. He put the body parts in bags and disposed of them in trash, assisted by an unwitting neighbour. Before going to KMA's home, Lewandowski left his details and address with Jacqueline Lewandowski her roommate (and cousin) who called the police next day when Ann Marie failed to return. Police searched MKA's premises and discovered the body parts in the trash.
References	Fox6News, 2018; Milwaukee County Case 2003CF001468; Vielmetti, 2018.

Peter Atkins, UK, 2001

Perpetrator	Peter Atkins, 48, male, white British, former garage owner, lived in Llandaff North, Cardiff, Wales.
P's mental health	PA had had schizophrenia for 18 years. In 1998, he had a relapse and had to give up work as a garage owner.

Victim	Stephen Provoost, 32, male, white British, social worker.
P–V relationship	PA was the victim's father-in-law.
Means	PA repeatedly stabbed the victim with a sheath knife killing him almost instantly from wounds to his neck, chest, and back.
Motive	PA told police of the killing, 'It did not seem real to me. It was like a dream'.
Opportunity	In the early hours of 25 January 2001 Atkins broke into his son-in-law and daughter's house, arming himself with a knife, and attacking Stephen Provoost in bed.
Location	The attack occurred at the house of Stephen Provoost and his wife Lisa (PA's daughter) in Rumney, Cardiff. PA drove to the Provoost house and broke in via the kitchen window. Entering the couple's bedroom, PA stabbed the victim who was in bed beside his wife Lisa (PA's daughter). Police arrested PA at the house.
Preventative strategy	Possible red flags were PA's accumulating problems. Following a heart attack, he became overly concerned about his health. He believed that his wife was having an affair and developed an animosity towards his son-in-law. In July 2000, PA after arguing with his daughter and her husband cut the petrol pipe on her car. A day before the killing, PA's wife Carol called police to visit their home fearing for her own safety. PA had punched her to the ground and then kicked her because the kitchen was messy. Also, greater home security for the house in Rumney, Cardiff may have prevented PA's entry.
Legal outcome	Convicted of manslaughter, PA was ordered to be detained in a high security psychiatric hospital.
References	BBC, 5 June 2001; BBC, 5 August 2019; Savill, 2001.

David Attias, USA, 2001

Perpetrator	David Attias, 18, male, white American, freshman at the University of California Santa Barbara (UCSB), son of a television director.
P's mental health	Before the killings, DA may have had mental health and drug problems.
Victims	Elie Israel, 27, a French native with a photography shop in San Francisco; Ruth Levy, 20, a student at Santa Barbara City College; Nicholas Bourdakis, 20, and Christopher Divis, 20, both UCSB students. All died before paramedics arrived.

P–V relationship	DA had no relationships with the victims.
Means	DA drove his Saab vehicle at speed into a group of young adults, killing four.
Motive	After killing, DA climbed on top of his vehicle declaring he was, 'the angel of death'. Blood tests indicated that DA was under the influence of marijuana and Lidocaine, but these were not deemed influential in the incident. After the murder conviction and before the insanity finding, DA's lawyer Jack Early reportedly said DA had been taking medication including 'at least one anti-psychotic' and had, 'no delusions, no psychosis now'. At Patton State Hospital DA was treated for bipolar disorder and pervasive developmental disorder.
Opportunity	The homicide occurred at 11 pm Friday 23 February 2001. The victims were walking by the road undefended, and DA drove the car at speed.
Location	The 6500 block of Sabado Tarde Road in the Isla Vista neighbourhood near UCSB.
Preventative strategy	Possibly better supervision given DA's apparent mental health and drug problems.
Legal outcome	At the 2002 trial DA was convicted of four counts of second-degree murder and acquitted of driving under the influence. A week later the same jury found DA legally insane. He was sent to a state mental institution Patton State Hospital, San Bernardino.
Notes	A civil lawsuit was brought by victims' parents against DA's parents for negligence on the grounds of allowing DA with known mental health and drug problems to have the car he used as a weapon.
References	Lagos, 2002; McKay, 2014; Sexton, 2001.

Marie Elise West, USA, 2000

Perpetrator	Marie Elise West, 35, female, white American with mixed race ancestry. Graduated UCLA in 1988 later enrolling as a law student at Boalt Hall law school, Berkley. She married three times. In 2000, living at Hermosa Beach, Los Angeles County, she worked at the Hermosa Steakout restaurant.
P's mental health	Soon after entering law school, MEW showed signs of mental disorder and was hospitalised for brief periods eventually leaving the school. MEW had been arrested six times and hospitalised 19 times since being diagnosed with 'bipolar disorder' in 1990. In 1993 she drove

her car into the Huntington Beach Pier believing that Nazis were gassing Jews beneath it. Two years later she attacked a teacher at an elementary school and, claiming she was the Messiah, warned students against being sold as sex slaves. Between 1990 and 2000 MEW tried law school three more times but withdrew after psychotic episodes. In March 2000, MEW was arrested for trespassing at a Redondo Beach hotel and hospitalised.

Victim	Jesus Plascencia, 65, male, American Latino, a Mexican immigrant, a busboy at Weiler's Deli.
P–V relationship	None.
Means	MEW repeatedly ran over the victim in her car.
Motive	Having run over the victim, MEW told a bagel shop employee that Plascencia was 'roadkill'.
Opportunity	The homicide occurred at 3.45 am 31 August 2000. The victim was walking unprotected, and MEW drove her car at him then over him before anyone could intervene.
Location	Van Nuys bagel shop parking lot, Los Angeles.
Preventative strategy	Hospitalisation may have been preventive. MEW had ten years of regular hospitalisation and on the night of the killings became out of control.
Legal outcome	In 2004 a jury found MEW guilty of second-degree murder and not guilty of a hate crime but disagreed whether she was sane. In 2006, a jury found MEW 'insane' and she was committed to a state psychiatric hospital.
Notes	On the evening of the killing, MEW's husband encouraged her to check in at Harbor-UCLA, but she declined. At the restaurant, MEW began acting erratically and was sent home. There she obsessed that Michael Maglieri, the son of a club owner, would be killed by gang members. At 11.30 pm she drove off in the car saying she would rescue Maglieri.
References	Clark, 2006; Teetor, 2002.

References

ABC News (updated 21 December 2014) 'Cairns woman charged with murder of eight children: Bodies found in Manoora house' ABC News. www.abc.net.au/news/2014-12-21/cairns-woman-charged-with-murder-of-eight-children/5981652.

Associated Press (23 November 2004 and 4 January 2015) *Cops: Mother cut off baby's arms' Fox News.* www.foxnews.com/story/cops-mother-cut-off-babys-arms.

Australian Associated Press (2017) 'Mother psychotic when she killed eight children, Queensland court rules' *The Guardian* (4 May 2017) www.theguardian.com/australia -news/2017/may/04/mother-psychotic-when-she-killed-eight-children-queensland-court -rules.

Baker, K. (2018) 'Why was mentally ill man set free to kill my husband?' *Mail Online* (2 July 2018) www.dailymail.co.uk/news/article-5909435/Psychotic-killer-stabbe d-renowned-academic-death-outside-home.html.

Barr, C. W., Londoño, E. and Morse, D. (2006) 'Patient admits killing psychiatrist, police say' *Washington Post* (5 September 2006) www.washingtonpost.com/wp-dyn/ content/article/2006/09/04/AR2006090400430.html.

BBC News (2001) 'Schizophrenic father detained for killing' BBC News (5 June 2001) http://news.bbc.co.uk/1/hi/wales/1371753.stm.

BBC News (2003) 'Mother and son killed by "psychotic"' BBC News (15 December 2003) http://news.bbc.co.uk/1/hi/england/beds/bucks/herts/3322525.stm.

BBC News (22 November 2011) 'Killings in Swindon by mental health patients "avoidable"' BBC News (22 November 2011) www.bbc.co.uk/news/uk-england-wilt shire-15834042.

BBC News (24 August 2011) 'Plan to free 'psychotic' double killer Gregory Davis' BBC (24 August 2011) www.bbc.co.uk/news/uk-england-beds-bucks-herts-14650739.

BBC (2013) 'Mental health review after Cray's Hill double death incident' BBC (27 March 2013) www. *bbc.co.uk/news/uk-england-essex*-21951670.

BBC News (2015) 'Manslaughter: Timothy Crook guilty of killing parents' BBC News (20 July 2015) www.*bbc.co.uk/news/uk-england-wiltshire*-33599525.

BBC News (2017) 'Mother 'not responsible' for killing eight children in Australia' BBC News (4 May 2017) www. *bbc.co.uk/news/world-australia*-39777191.

BBC News (2018) 'Jeroen Ensink inquest: Killer's sister had warned police' BBC News (3 July 2018) www. *bbc.co.uk/news/uk-england-london*-44693781.

BBC News (2019) 'Killer Peter Atkins missing from secure hospital' BBC News (5 August 2019) www. *bbc.co.uk/news/uk-england-cambridgeshire*-49234684.

Bernstein, E. and Koppel. N. (2008) 'A Death in the Family’ *Wall Street Journal* (16 August 2008) www.wsj.com/articles/SB121883750650245525.

Bhogal, K. (2017) *An Independent Investigation into the Care and Treatment of P in the West Midlands.* Niche Health and Social Care Consulting (14 June 2017) www. england.nhs.uk/midlands/wp-content/uploads/sites/46/2019/05/independent-investiga tion-care-treatment-patient-p.pdf.

Boston News (2006) 'Mentally ill son charged with murdering his mother' *Boston News* (22 June 2006) http://archive.boston.com/news/local/maine/articles/2006/06/ 22/mentally_ill_soncharged_with_murdering_his_mother/.

Celona, L. and Golding, B. (2017) 'NYPD cop-killer was a schizophrenic off his meds: Girlfriend' *New York Post* (5 July 2017) https://nypost.com/2017/07/05/nypd-cop -killer-was-a-schizophrenic-off-his-meds-girlfriend/.

Clark, S. (2006) 'Jury finds killer was insane' *Los Angeles Times* (16 August 2006) www.latimes.com/archives/la-xpm-2006-aug-16-me-west16-story.html.

Cleary, T. (2017) 'Alexander Bonds: Five fast facts you need to know' *Heavy.com* (5 July 2017) https://heavy.com/news/2017/07/john-alexander-bonds-nypd-officer-cop -shot-killed-suspect-photos-ambush-attack/.

CNN/KLTV (2003) 'Texas woman, Member of Assembly of God, says God Told her to Kill Sons' *Internet Archive* (13 May 2003) www.cephas-library.com/assembly_of_god/assembly_of_god_member_killed_her_sons.html.

Davies, C. (2018a) '"They're coming to get me": Troubled student who killed an academic' *The Guardian* (17 July 2018) www.theguardian.com/uk-news/2018/jul/17/femi-nandap-troubled-student-killed-academic.

Davies, C. (2018b) 'Inquest criticises police over London killing of Dutch academic' *The Guardian* (17 July 2018) www.theguardian.com/uk-news/2018/jul/17/inquest-criticises-police-over-london-killing-of-dutch-academic-jeroen-ensink.

Dilley, S. and Kemp, P. (2019) Alexander-Lewis Ranwell: The triple killer who was arrested twice BBC News (2 December 2019) www. *bbc.co.uk/news/uk-england-devon*-50591491.

Docking, N. (21 December 2018) 'Man stabbed his mum to death and tried to kill his gran's carer in psychotic episode’ *Echo* (21 December 2018) www.liverpoolecho.co.uk/news/liverpool-news/christian-lacey-liz-lacey-murder–15584632.

Dolan, A. (2009) 'Young mother stabbed to death after police ignored warning that killer father posed threat' *The Daily Mail* (6 October 2009) www.dailymail.co.uk/news/article-1218528/Young-mother-stabbed-death-police-ignored-warning-killer-posed-threat.html.

Ellis, T. M. and Emily, J. (2006) 'Child-killer to leave hospital' *The Dallas Morning News* (10 November 2006) www.pressreader.com/usa/the-dallas-morning-news/20061110/281552286359490.

Evans, M. (2018) 'Widow of academic stabbed to death on his doorstep demands to know why psychotic knifeman was released to kill' *Telegraph* (2 July 2018) www.telegraph.co.uk/news/2018/07/02/psychotic-killer-attacked-new-father-told-police-leave-dead/.

Falkenberg, L. (2003) 'Closing arguments begin in Texas mother's murder trial' Associated Press (3 April 2003) www.cephas-library.com/assembly_of_god/assembly_of_god_member_killed_her_sons.html.

Ferris, I. (2015) 'Man with schizophrenia who murdered his parents detained for life' *Mirror* (29 July 2015) www.mirror.co.uk/news/uk-news/man-paranoid-schizophrenia-who-murdered–6160165.

News (2018) 'Man who killed teen, dismembered her body could be released from mental health facility soon' www.dailymotion.com/video/x6hmen7.

Gilligan, A. (2013) 'Truth about dangerous mental patients let out to kill' *The Telegraph* (5 October 2013) www.telegraph.co.uk/news/uknews/crime/10358251/Truth-about-dangerous-mental-patients-let-out-to-kill.html.

Heart Radio (no date) 'Essex: Family tribute after two shot' Heart Radio. www.heart.co.uk/essex/news/local/essex-family-tribute-after-two-shot/.

Hinman, M. (2018) 'Familia earns NYPD's medal of honor' *The Riverdale Press* (7 July 2018) https://riverdalepress.com/stories/familia-earns-nypds-medal-of-honor,66150.

Humphries, J. (2019) 'Son's brutal killing of mum could have been avoided if not for "deadly errors"' *Mirror* (27 May 2019) www.mirror.co.uk/news/uk-news/sons-brutal-killing-mum-could–16208553.

Joyner, J. (2004) 'Mom cut off baby's arms' *Outside the Beltway* (23 November 2004) www.outsidethebeltway.com/mom_cut_off_babys_arms/.

Lagos, M. (2002) 'Jury finds Attias guilty of murder' *Daily Nexus* (6 June 2002) http://dailynexus.com/2002-06-06/jury-finds-attias-guilty-of-murder/.

Maynaya, E. (2016) 'She repeated to me, "I am afraid dad"' *Gazeta.ru* (3 February 2016) www.gazeta.ru/politics/2016/03/02_a_8105087.shtml.

McKay, H. (2014) ''01 Santa Barbara killer walks free as families relive carnage 13 years later' Fox News (30 May 2014 updated 20 November 2015) www.foxnews.com/us/01-santa-barbara-killer-walks-free-as-families-relive-carnage-13-years-later.

Middleton, J. (2019) 'Too middle class to kill: Son with schizophrenia was left to stab his mother to death as doctors and police thought he was too well-healed to be dangerous' *Mail Online* (27 May 2019) www.dailymail.co.uk/news/article-7074549/Police-medics-missed-two-chances-stop-mentally-ill-man-killing-mother-report-finds.html.

Milwaukee County Case 2003CF001468 *State of Wisconsin vs. Keith Michael Addy* https://wcca.wicourts.gov/caseDetail.html?cacheId=19D57A47CFCA121AB4538508BF3315A7&caseNo=2003CF001468&countyNo=40&mode=details&offset=11&recordCount=12#summary.

Morris, S. (2019) 'Killer of three elderly Devon men found not guilty of murder due to insanity' *The Guardian* (2 December 2019) www.theguardian.com/uk-news/2019/dec/02/killer-of-three-elderly-devon-men-found-not-guilty-due-to-insanity.

NHS England (2013) *Report to NHS England of the Independent Investigation into the Healthcare and Treatment of 'Patient P'* (Commissioned by the Former North East Strategic Health Authority) http://hundredfamilies.org/wp/wp-content/uploads/2013/12/RONALD_DIXON_May06.pdf.

Nolan, S. (2013) 'Grieving sister accuses mental health doctors of failing her family after "dangerous and psychotic" brother shot their mother then killed himself' *Mail Online* (28 March 2013) www.dailymail.co.uk/news/article-2300652/Grieving-sister-accuses-mental-health-doctors-failing-family-dangerous-psychotic-brother-shot-mother-killed-himself.html.

North Wales Live (2013) 'Was killer given the care that he needed while in North Wales?' North Wales Live (13 May 2013) www. *dailypost.co.uk/news/north-wales-news/deyan-deyanov-killer-given-care*-3661581.

Novacic, I. (2015) *'Violent minds: Standing at the crossroads of mental health, public safety'* CBS News (16 June 2015) www.cbsnews.com/news/violent-minds-standing-at-the-crossroads-of-mental-health-public-safety/.

Porter, M. (2015) 'Addict who killed his mum funded heroin addiction after her football pools jackpot' *Echo* (26 November 2015) www.echo-news.co.uk/news/14103269.addict-who-killed-his-mum-funded-heroin-habit-after-her-football-pools-jackpot/.

Prendergast, D. and Sheehan, K. (2017) 'NYPD cop assassin was a drifter who once beat up an officer' *New York Post* (5 July 2017) https://nypost.com/2017/07/05/nypd-cop-assassin-was-a-drifter-who-once-beat-up-an-officer/.

Reed, A. (2014) *Homicide Investigation Report into the Death of a Child* Strategic Executive Information System (STEIS) Reference 2013/7122. www.hundredfamilies.org/wp/wp-content/uploads/2014/10/PHILLIP_SIMELANEMar13_FULL.pdf.

Religion News Blog (2008) 'Dean Schlosser who cut off baby's arms moving to outpatient care' *Religion News Blog* (12 November 2008) www.religionnewsblog.com/22921/dena-schlosser.

Reporter (3 April 2006) 'Paranoid schizophrenic Marc Carter jailed for Bristol Samurai sword killing of Gino Nelmes' *HuffPost* (1 February 2013 and updated 3 April 2013) www.huffingtonpost.co.uk/2013/02/01/pranoid-schizophrenic-man2599343.html.

Reporter (16 May 2007) 'Son faces grand jury in mother's murder' *The Connection* (16 May 2007) www.connectionnewspapers.com/news/2007/may/16/son-faces-grand-jur y-in-mothers-murder/.

Reporter (2 August 2007) 'Schizophrenic addicted to skunk cannabis killed best friend' *Evening Standard* (2 August 2007) www.standard.co.uk/news/schizophrenic-addic ted-to-skunk-cannabis-killed-best-friend-6602755.html.

Reporter (18 December 2007) 'Jones found not guilty by reason of insanity' *The Connection* (18 December 2007) www.connectionnewspapers.com/news/2007/dec/18/ jones-not-guilty-by-reason-of-insanity/.

Reporter (18 September 2012) 'Gino Nelmes sword killing: Marc Carter admits man-slaughter' BBC (18 September 2012) www.bbc.co.uk/news/uk-england-bristol– 19640622.

Reporter (2 October 2013) 'Christina Edkins' killing: Philip Simelane detained' BBC News (2 October 2013) www.bbc.co.uk/news/uk-england-birmingham–24358473.

Reporter (4 March 2016) 'Nanny Charged with Murder of 4-year Old Child in Moscow' *The Moscow Times* (4 March 2016) www.themoscowtimes.com/2016/03/ 04/nanny-charged-with-murder-of-4-year-old-child-in-moscow-a52076.

Reporter (11 March 2016) 'Moscow nanny says 'voices' told her to commit murder' *The Moscow Times* (11 March 2016) www.themoscowtimes.com/2016/03/11/m oscow-nanny-says-voices-told-her-to-commit-murder-a52134.

Reporter (27 April 2016) 'Moscow nanny charged with beheading child sent to psy-chiatric prison' *The Moscow Times* (27 April 2016) www.themoscowtimes.com/2016/ 04/27/moscow-nanny-charged-with-beheading-child-sent-to-psychiatric-prison-a52700.

riafan.ru (2016) 'Killer nanny strangled the girl before cutting off her head' *riafan.ru* (29 February 2016) https://riafan.ru/506049-nyanya-ubiica-zadushila-devochku-pered-tem-kak-otrezat-ei-golovu.

Robinson, S. (2013) 'Paranoid schizophrenic with history of "extreme violence" stabbed man 17 times' *Mail Online* (1 February 2013) www.dailymail.co.uk/news/article-2272072/Samurai-sword-murder-Paranoid-schizophrenic-Marc-Carter-stabbed-Gino-Nelmes-17-times.html.

Savill, R. (2001) 'Son-in-law stabbed to death in marital bed’ *The Telegraph* (6 June 2001) www.telegraph.co.uk/news/uknews/1311615/Son-in-law-stabbed-to-dea th-in-marital-bed.html.

Scott, S. (2013) 'Revealed: Inside the mind of paranoid knifeman Ronald Dixon' *Newcastle Chronicle/Chronicle Live* (30 May 2013) www.chroniclelive.co.uk/news/ north-east-news/revealed-inside-mind-paranoid-knifeman–4029701.

Sexton, S. (2001) 'UCSB student kills four in high speed crash' *The Daily Californian* (26 February 2001) https://archive.dailycal.org/article.php?id=4694.

Simon, R. I. (2011) 'Patient violence against healthcare professionals' *Psychiatric Times 28, 2* (3 March 2011) www.psychiatrictimes.com/psychiatric-emergencies/pa tient-violence-against-health-care-professionals.

Sky News (2013) 'Tenerife beheading: Killer gets 20 years' Sky News (28 February 2013) https://news.sky.com/story/tenerife-beheading-killer-gets-20-years–10453185.

Sky News (2019) 'Paranoid schizophrenic Alexander Lewis-Ranwell not guilty of murder-ing three pensioners' Sky News (2 December 2019) https://news. *sky.com/story/paranoid-schizophrenic-man-not-guilty-of-murderers-three-pensioners-hours-apart-*11876554.

TASS (2016) 'The murder of a child in Moscow: Investigation progress and public reaction' TASS (29 February 2016) https://tass.ru/proisshestviya/2706157 (in Russian).

Teetor, P. (2002) 'Prelude to a death' *Los Angeles Times* (5 May 2002) www.latimes.com/archives/la-xpm-2002-may-05-tm-41435-story.html.

Twomey, J. (2009) 'Fury after psychotic killer walks free after four years' *Express* (22 April 2002) www.express.co.uk/news/uk/96406/Fury-as-psychotic-killer-walks-free-after-4-years.

Vielmetti, B. (2018) 'Man who killed, dismembered woman denied release from mental hospital' *Milwaukee Journal Sentinel* (16 April 2018) https://eu.jsonline.com/story/news/crime/2018/04/12/man-who-killed-dismembered-woman-2003-denied-release-mental-hospital/511533002/.

Welton, B. (2013) 'Birmingham bus killer Philip Simelane to be held at a psychiatric unit indefinitely' *Manchester Evening News* (2 October 2013) www.manchestereveningnews.co.uk/news/uk-news/birmingham-bus-killer-phillip-simelane–6128265.

Whitley, G. (2005) 'Psycho Mom' *Dallas Observer* (20 January 2005) www.dallasobserver.com/news/psycho-mom–6408764.

Wiggin, K. (2011) 'Patient who killed psychiatrist now accused of slaying hospital roommate' CBS News (24 October 2011) www.cbsnews.com/news/patient-who-killed-psychiatrist-now-accused-of-slaying-hospital-roommate/.

Wiles, D. (2013) 'Criticism of mental health unit in charge of killer Michael Harris' *Swindon Advertiser* (9 February 2013).

Index

Note: Page numbers in **bold** indicate text contained within tables.

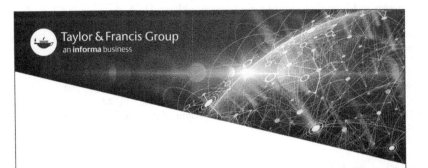

For Product Safety Concerns and Information please contact our EU representative GPSR@taylorandfrancis.com Taylor & Francis Verlag GmbH, Kaufingerstraße 24, 80331 München, Germany

Printed and bound by CPI Group (UK) Ltd, Croydon, CR0 4YY
08/06/2025
01897007-0008